The Encyclopedia of ATHLETIC MEDICINE

by Dr. George Sheehan

Drawings by Bil Canfield

IBSN: 0-89037-015-X

Eleventh Printing, May 1980

ANDERSON WORLD, INC.
Box 159, Mountain View, CA 94042

CONTENTS

(**Note:** "Ailments—'A' to 'Z' " on page 95 is an index on information on specific illnesses and injuries. Refer to it for page numbers.)

FOREWORD

George Sheehan is eminently qualified to compile this booklet. He's a medical doctor and a professional writer. And he's more than that. Dr. Sheehan is a runner—everything from mile to marathon—who has felt the pains of the sport as well as treated them. This gives him special insight.

The New Jersey internist, who writes for *Runner's World* and other publications, looks at sports medicine from the runner's viewpoint. He realizes that running injuries are subtle, and that "quit running" is the worst medical advice a runner can hear. He knows that it takes a special kind of doctor to treat the healthiest people in the society instead of the unhealthiest, and that plain health—the mere absence of disease—and a fine edge of fitness are entirely different things.

Preventive medicine occupies Dr. Sheehan's attention. He's more interested in blocking illness and injury at the source than in picking up doctor's fees for treating symptoms. He knows from painful personal experience the disruption these things cause.

Unfortunately, he knows too that running is a high-stress activity, and the odds indicate that every runner is likely to be temporarily disabled perhaps once a year.

It doesn't take much to throw a finely-tuned runner out of whack, and out of competition. A cold here, a blister there. A sore knee, a tender tendon, an upset stomach. Things that would hardly be noticed by the man in his easy chair are disastrous to the runner on the road or track.

This is the paradox of running, and the key problem in running medicine. The harder a runner works at getting fit, the more likely he'll encounter ailments that destroy his fitness. Overwork, Sheehan says, leads to most running breakdowns. Gaining fitness is a process of adapting to stress, but too much stress leads to injuries and illnesses. The problem is finding the balance.

Throughout this booklet, there is considerable emphasis on finding and keeping this crucial balance between necessary stress and overstressing—which is also the difference between hard, rewarding work and hard, killing work. The inner ecology is balanced delicately.

This is the first booklet of its type, specializing on the ailments of runners. Dr. Sheehan and his assistants have written a complete guide on the subject. It is meant to help runners understand what ails them. Much of the material is unconventional by established medical standards. But remember that runners are somewhat unconventional, too, and established medical practices haven't always worked for them.

New and sometimes revolutionary treatment methods are coming out of running. Many of the new practices here are still theories—tested theories, but still not accepted medical practice. Some of these are controversial. Keep this warning in mind as you read.

Remember, too, that this booklet is not intended specifically to diagnose individual cases. Runners should consult their own doctors on all serious health questions. A faulty self-diagnosis at best will slow recovery; at worst it can threaten all future running.

Chapter One

Causes and Prevention

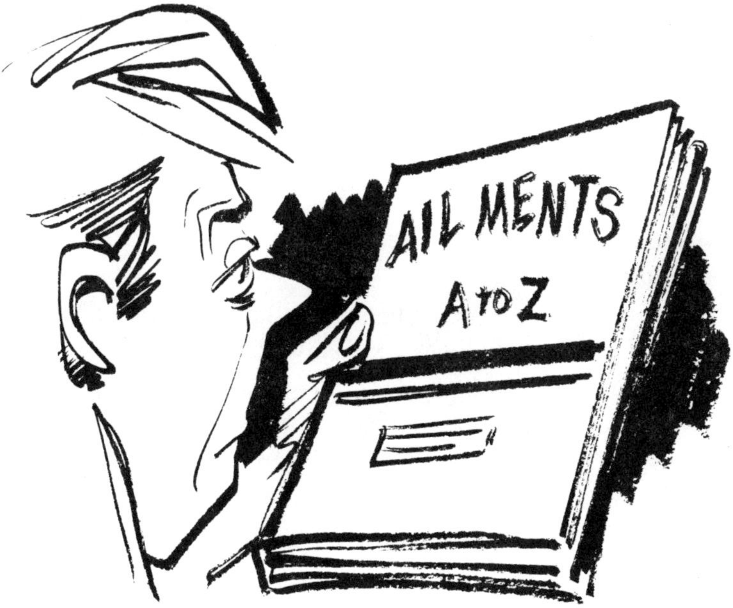

INTRODUCTION

This chapter stresses the general principles of athletic medicine. General articles—and the specific ones that follow—make sense only if they emphasize these underlying principles. Those few we have should be emphasized.

- Sports medicine is in its infancy. What you are about to read is 50% fact, and we're not sure which 50% that is.

- The diseases of athletes are diseases of overuse: too much training plus a susceptible individual. When you overwork, you break down at your weakest point. Train, don't strain.

- The diseases of athletes are subtle, and not easily detected and treated—even by medical professionals. Unconventional treatment is often called for.

- The pursuit of excellence requires cooperation with personal body rhythms and individual strengths and weaknesses. We must cooperate with nature, not assault it.

- Each of us is an experiment-of-one, seeking to discover more and more about the exquisite design and capabilities of our human body.

- The aim of sports medicine is to keep the athlete active, and free to climb to the peak of his physical potential.

This chapter—in fact, this entire booklet—emphasizes the root causes of athletic ailments. Understanding these causes will help the athlete stop injuries and illnesses at the source—BEFORE they require medical attention. Preventive medicine is far more conducive than "patch-up-and-repair" to good health and consistent high-level running performance.

THE HEALTHY APPROACH

BY GEORGE SHEEHAN, M.D.

The athlete has brought a new dimension to medicine.

Health.

Medicine has too long concerned itself with the treatment of disease and has considered the absence of disease to be health. But now the athlete has provided medicine with the *New Normal*—man at his maximum; his muscular, metabolic, physiological, cardio-pulmonary and psychological maximum.

How to reach that maximum is as much a part of this book as the treatment of ailments along the way. Finding one's peak steady state—and keeping it—is no easy task. Nature does not give up her secrets willingly. The athlete must be always on the alert to learn about his body and its uniqueness. That is a key principle—the uniqueness of each athlete in his reaction to effort and strain and stress.

What this means is that training (and that includes sleep, diet, practice time, duration and activity, and relaxation) must be tailored to each individual. The program should fit *you,* not the other way around. When you deviate from what is best for you, you will hear about it in some way: a pain here, a soreness there, respiratory infection, a bad performance, some physical or mental change.

These are the signs and symptoms of overuse. This might truly be called a book of overuse diseases—illnesses developing from pushing yourself beyond the capabilities of your constitution.

However, since we are aware of where most of these breakdowns occur, and why, the athlete can make a personal assessment prior to beginning training which can be quite valuable.

• First and foremost would be to analyze your feet. The fact that you have never had foot trouble before means nothing. As soon as the distances begin to increase, hidden weaknesses can cause major trouble. A second toe that is longer than the first toe is one sign of a structural weakness that can give trouble later on. A very high arch is another anatomical variation that can lead to difficulties.

• The leg muscles come next. Tightness of the hamstrings, the large muscles on the back of the thigh, suggest future problems with achilles tendonitis, low back or sciatic pain. Efforts should be made to loosen them by flexibility exercises, going barefoot, and exercising foot, shin and quadriceps muscles may be necessary.

• Lordosis, or sway back, is another potentially incapacitating disorder. Every effort should be made to strengthen and straighten the back. The exercise with weights of the opposing muscles (in this case the stomach) is something that should be done for all muscle groups, including leg, thigh and shoulders.

• Other systems besides the muscular ones can break down under stress. Care should be taken that the athlete gets enough sleep. Too much sleep at one time, however, can do as much harm as too little. A person's sleep requirements are highly individualistic and should be adhered to. If sleep is lost, it might better be made up in a nap during the day than increasing the the night's span.

- There is little place in the athlete's diet for sweets and extra calories. Even 10 miles a day allows him only an extra 1000. The less he weighs, as long as his lean muscle mass is unaffected, the better will be his performance. Almost all of us eat too much. Man was constructed so that he could go for long periods without normal food intake; he was not, and is not, ready for the overfeeding we get today.

Even with optimum diet, sleep, muscle development and with preventive foot care, the athlete must still assess himself in several ways to prevent disaster. First, he must tune in on his body rhythms and get to know himself better; recognize how much work he can handle.

Has he always been a bull for work or does he tire easily? Does his body take a long time to recoup from loss of sleep, exposure to chilling and rain? If so, he may find that he will have to intersperse his rigorous training days with one or two easy ones.

He should also know whether he is a day or night person. Should he do most of his training at certain times of the day? This decision may be crucial in the persistence of his daily workouts.

In the following pages we will be presenting the consequences of the enormous training loads of today's athletes on their feet, knees, thighs and backs, as well as their gastro-intestinal, circulatory, pulmonary, urological, endocrine, hematologic and nervous systems. We are pursuing excellence. And, unfortunately, when the athlete is at his peak he is also just a hair's breadth away from being overtrained, and therefore susceptible to many of the symptoms described.

The recent *Encyclopedia of Sports Medicine* was said by the editor to contain only about 50% fact; the rest was speculation. I don't think he exaggerated. But we are in a continuing dialogue and feedback so that the runners themselves are gradually coming up with solutions to the problems. What we present here may well change in the next 12 months. Many of my past answers to medical questions in *Runner's World* would now be different. And this is because the runners have persisted and discovered, on their own, clues that have led to new and better ideas in treatment and diagnosis.

We urge you to join this crusade for health.

ADAPTING TO STRESSES

A basis for modern athletic training is the General Adaptation Syndrome (GAS) theory developed by Canadian physiologist Hans Selye.

In simplest terms, Selye's theory says that a person exposed to stress (running is one stress among many) throws up defenses to counteract it. If the stress is applied in small enough quantities and regularly enough, the body adapts to it. But if the doses are too heavy, the body can't cope. It goes into the "exhaustion" phase of the syndrome, becoming highly susceptible to a number of stress ailments. These include ulcers, migraine, mental disorders, heart disease and the like.

The trick in running training is to train enough to build, but not so much that you tear down. The same exercise does both. Amount and pace makes the difference. The runner stays on a thin line between the two, and it's said that when he's in peak condition, he's just a step away from "exhaustion."

As the runner approaches the "exhausted" state, his body and mind give off a number of preliminary warning signals. These include persistent soreness and stiffness, nervousness, unexplained drops in performance and many others. (The symptoms are explored fully in the article "Reading Body Signs.")

The runner, in short, faces the dilemma of applying enough stress to get himself fit, but at the same time maintaining a reservoir of freshness, sharpness and eagerness which allows him to meet emergencies.

Reference: *Joe Henderson, Runner's World, September 1971.*

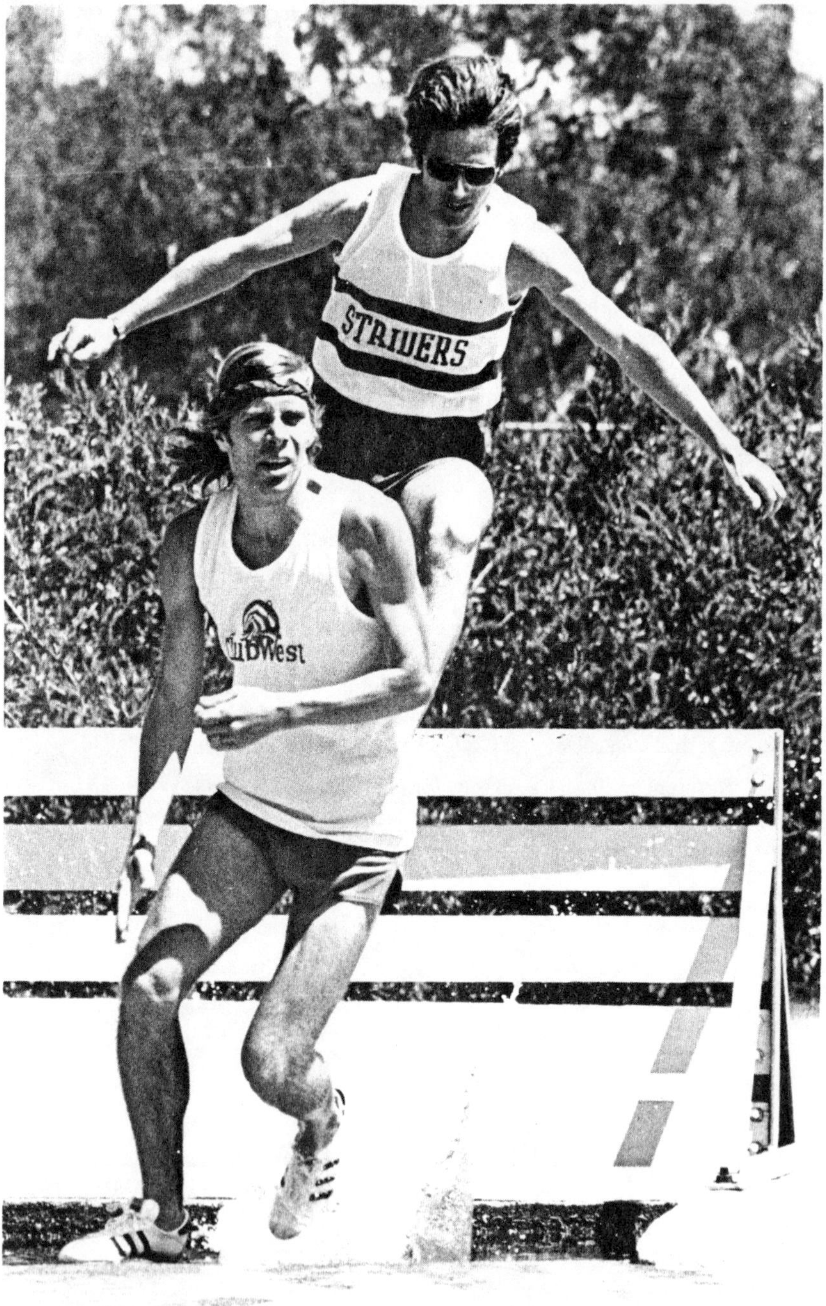

The risky impact of steeplechasing. (Stan Pantovic photo)

WORKING AWAY HEALTH

"Give Americans Wednesdays off!"

That's my suggestion to the Senators who passed the $1.47-billion bill intended to find a cure to the epidemic of heart disease in the United States.

"Work is the cause of our heart attacks!"

That's my word to the researchers who will man the 10 heart disease prevention centers and the 30 basic research centers the money will build and staff.

Forget about obesity, high cholesterol and excessive smoking. They are simply friends of the killer, incidental to the addiction Americans have for work.

Work is the real killer. It provides the stress. And coronary disease is a stress disease. Like ulcers and colitis and nervous breakdowns, it results from an overload—either physical, mental or psychological, or combinations of all three. The patient, in effect, blows a fuse. Work usually supplies the decisive amount of stress.

Work remains the main source of stress in a person's life (unless he has opted for the greater stress of disability, prolonged education, or welfare). It also remains for most of us a satisfying and important human activity. There and there alone can many of us find creativity, self-expression, self-esteem and feelings of security. Work, said Freud, is essential to mental health. It absorbs, he claimed, hostility and aggression. Work also satisfies our need to be with people; to participate and know our participation is valued; to contribute and know we are contributing.

The psychologists have told us about these good things, and I believe them. They have analyzed and reanalyzed work, looking for ways to provide involvement and satisfaction and psychological growth. They have introduced techniques to make people feel responsible and wanted and important.

But they forget one thing. We are bodies. They tend to forget about a man's guts, to ignore his heart and arteries and his colon and duodenal bulb. They need to be reminded that a man's internal milieu, that miraculous balance of water and salts and hormones, is as much at issue as his psychological adjustment.

Optimum work conditions must include an optimum work day and optimum work week. Sooner or later physiologists will know how to measure the effects of stress on the various systems of the body. Sooner or later, we will be told the ideal work day and the ideal work week, and that it varies from person to person

This ideal schedule, it seems to me, will have not more than two—certainly no more than three—work days in a row. There are few members of the population who can put four hard days in succession, much less five. On the fifth day or possibly the fourth, work which exists for man's survival becomes a killer. That is the crux of the situation.

Take the athlete. He often bases his training schedule on the hard-day/easy-day routine. Some might run two hard days and then the easy day which may be hardly more than working up a sweat. Even ultra-long distance runners, the 50-milers, take two days a week where they jog lightly.

The athlete knows that when stress is applied the body must be given a chance to recoup. The worker's stress is different, but aggravation and tension and frustration add up like miles on a track. And five or four or even three of these days can be much too much.

That's where Wednesday comes in—a day to adapt, a day to meditate. Sunday is for God. Saturday is for play. Wednesday is for self. Wednesday puts the rest of the week, even the rest of your life, in perspective. Used for reading, self-improvement or simply contemplating the sky, it tells you what your job really means and where it fits in the scheme of things.

The best method of coping with stress is in the rest and self-expression only Wednesday can bring: that special sanity that comes in the middle of the week whan man can stand back from God and country and family and work, and for 24 hours just be himself. *(BY GEORGE SHEEHAN, M.D.)*

Next Page: The marathoner's feet and legs absorb tens of thousands of individual road shocks during the course of the race. The stress takes a high toll. (Don Chadez photo)

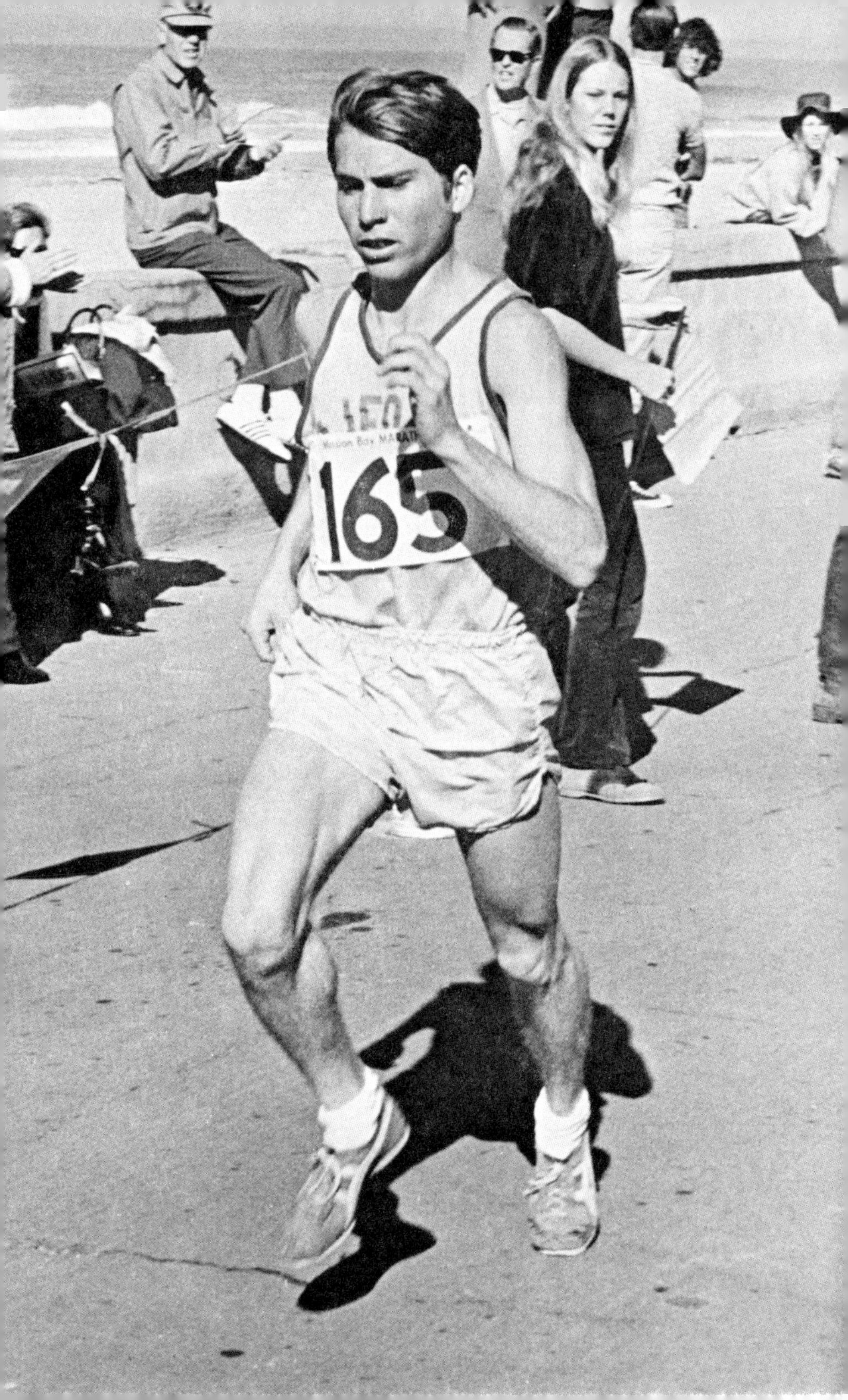
165

READING BODY SIGNS

Ecology begins at home. Inside each of us is an ecological system as intricate and marvelously balanced as any system outside. Once we learn the importance of living in harmony with ourselves, we'll become more sensitive to the harmony and balance of the outer environment.

"Inner-ecology" is a blending of life forces that ebb and flow programmed patterns. When the individual parts are meshing properly, we have health, fitness and good performance. But when one part of the system acts up, there is chaos because the fine balance has been destroyed.

The human body/mind is a symphony. Some of the individual instruments are booming, some are whispering, making melodies, harmonies and rhythms. When the individual parts are blending as intended, you don't hear individual parts. You hear the musical whole, and it's beautiful. But a single instrument out of tune can destroy the music, and make you painfully aware of the discord. The entire symphony is thrown off.

We have a symphony of signs that tell us when we're in tune or out. It's a wise runner who develops a sensitive ear for the body's notes. By reading and interpreting these signs, he can go a long way toward stopping trouble at its source.

All stress injuries and illnesses give advance warning before they strike. These things don't happen at random, without cause or reason, and athletic ailments aren't mysterious, fateful happenings. Their histories are easily traced–usually resulting from (1) overwork, combined with (2) refusing to heed mild preliminary warning symptoms.

It's as simple as this: When we run too far and too fast, too often, we get sore and tired. Nature is showing us we've thrown ourselves out of tune by producing mild pain and fatigue. She's saying, "Slow down, my friend." These warnings are for our protection. The unpleasantness disappears once the balance is restored. Keep fighting it, though, and it escalates into real trouble.

Fighting or ignoring instinctive "body wisdom" may give apparent victories. But they are only temporary. This is installment-plan living–buy now, pay later–and the bill will eventually come due. For every day a man fails to heed nature's friendly little reminders, a bit more is added to tomorrow's bill. As the bill adds up, the reminders get progressively less friendly.

Listen to the inner symphony with a keen ear. The key players can be divided into two groups.

OBJECTIVE SIGNS– The measurable ones include performance, weight, pulse, breathing, elimination and sleep. Like all body actions, they operate on fairly steady schedules. Keep tuned in for sudden, drastic changes from the norms.

- **Performance**–Sudden drops in the ability to handle distances or paces.
- **Weight**–Drastic drops in weight–say, several pounds in a day or two.
- **Pulse**–Significant increases in normal resting rate.

• **Breathing**—Anaerobic (forced breathing) running begins at a considerably slower pace than normal.

• **Elimination**—Any major deviation from normal schedule of urination and defecation.

• **Sleep**—Extreme difficulty in getting to sleep, or staying asleep (particularly the latter).

SUBJECTIVE SIGNS— These are best described as "feelings" that things inside aren't quite right. They include pain, illness, fatigue, appetite, thirst and "psychological resilience."

• **Pain**—Perhaps the single most important warning sign. Pains in the muscles, joints and tendons are the most common. Pains that increase while running are more serious than those which gradually diminish in the course of the run.

• **Illness**—Frequent colds, sore throats, headaches, and stomach upsets.

• **Fatigue**—Nagging tiredness that lingers long after runs are completed, and carries over from day to day.

• **Appetite**—Disinterest in eating.

• **Thirst**—Insatiable craving for liquids, which is often a sign of chronic dehydration.

• **Psychological Resilience**—A mixed bag of symptoms including lack of enthusiasm or confidence, inability to relax, irritability, etc.

A final note to sensitive listeners to the body's sympony:

Your entire life style—with its multiple stresses—must be taken into account when you're monitoring and interpreting signs. Running is but one of many forces at work. Employment, family and social situations and the physical environment all add their load in stress. Getting in harmony in your running only takes you part way toward ecological living.

MILEAGE MANIA'S COST

BY CLIFF TEMPLE

Temple is the track and field writer for the Sunday Times of London. This article is reprinted with permission of that newspaper.

Sometimes when training in Ron Clarke's Australian tracksuit, given to him as a present, Dick Taylor says: "By golly, the old tracksuit's going fast today. Can't keep up with it."

Now other top runners are finding a similar problem: their legs won't keep up with the spiraling amount of training being demanded of them. While half the nation settles down for a lethargic evening in front of the box, the international runner is putting on his training shoes, damp from earlier exertions, often for the second or third time that day.

The momentum becomes obsessional. A delay at an airport becomes "time for a quick one," with steaming bodies padding through the departure lounge. Dave Bedford trains three times on the day before the international cross-country championship, though he knows he should be storing up energy. But he still wins, and the perpetual motion theory is strengthened.

"One of the penalties for higher performance levels involving such frequent training, near the athlete's physical limit, is an increased rate of breakdown through injury," says Dr. Peter Sperryn, honorary medical officer to the British Amateur Athletic Board. He's seriously alarmed at the number of distance runners he's had to treat recently.

Like advertisers crawling over each other to produce bigger–and therefore better–goods, some distance runners may become the fittest group of athletes ever to miss the Olympic Games through injury. For, inadvertently, applying the Peter Principle to athletics, they climb the ladder of quantity training until they reach the level of muscular incompetence. Then fibers rebel.

"There are three types of sporting injuries," says Dr. Sperryn. "Direct injuries, such as a fracture or concussion; indirect injuries, caused by violent forces not involving physical contact, such as sprains and muscle tears; and overuse injuries, incurred through excessive repetitive movements in training and competition.

"Out of 49 cases I have dealt with recently among middle-distance runners, 71% had overuse injuries, mainly in the Achilles tendon."

The best way to incense any distance runner is to ask if he's going out to "practice." The implication that he has not yet mastered the difficult business of placing one foot in front of the other is sufficient to annoy anyone who, in training, does precious little else six or seven million times a year.

Or eight million. The currency of distance running is "miles per week," and forever being devalued. Fifteen years ago, training meant going out five or six times a week, usually after work. Total: 60 miles, maybe 70. Today 100 miles a week, or around 15 miles a day, is looked on as fairly ordinary. Dave Bedford runs twice that much, usually training three times a day. It is said he once met himself coming back from the previous session.

"In running even 100 miles a week," explains Dr. Sperryn, "the athlete plants his foot on the ground not less than three million times during a year.

On each step, the muscle must not only project but also absorb the shock of impact. Injuries would be reduced if athletes would run more on grass, and in padded shoes. Most hammer out their training on roads without adequate protection against jarring.

The big question mark on their competitive improvement now is simply whether they can keep free of injury.

"I want athletes to stop and think about what they're doing. I've got the greatest respect for Bedford, who's built up carefully to his current intensive training. It's his imitators I'm more concerned about. The boys have got the mileage bug. Because they read Bedford is doing 200 miles a week, they're pushing their own training up far too quickly. They're just not thinking. There's no logical stop. They just keep in piling up the miles until they get injured. And that seems to be the sole limiting factor."

But if future distance runners are going to break the records Bedford has and will set, the question is how. Will they have to top his highest week's mileage of 235, or over 32 miles a day?

No, says Dr. Sperryn. "There must be some optimum point at which the body rebels. Already we have heard of athletes suffering dehydration and kidney trouble from trying to maintain their high weekly mileage.

"I think athletes must look more closely at what they're trying to achieve. Very few actually train much at or above racing pace. They do long, slow distance work and expect speed will follow automatically. But why? I think a smaller amount of more concentrated effort would not only produce better results, it would also cut down a lot of these injuries."

AVOIDING ALL INJURIES

BY TOM OSLER

Tom Osler, a college mathematics professor, is author of the booklet "Conditioning of Distance Runners." Here he expands on some of the ideas presented in that valuable work.

INTRODUCTION

The purpose of this article is to discuss, in practical terms, the nature, detection and prevention of overstress from distance running. I confess a certain missionary zeal in preparing these words, for after 18 years of running I feel that most runners I have met would do well to contemplate this most important subject.

The material which follows was learned through trial and error. The first 10 years of my running (ages 14-24) left me with injuries of the achilles tendons, arches and knees. Also, my racing performances were very unpredictable. Repetition of a particular training method could not guarantee repetition of racing times. Ten years of running had taught me nothing.

Finally, a severe injury of the hip left me feeling that I might never recover, and in this atmosphere of frustration I decided to "run for fun" and forget serious racing. Away went words like "strain against pain," and "the harder you work, the better you get," which I had trusted so long. In place of the previous hard discipline, I substituted slow, painless running.

Naturally, I expected my performances would gradually decline, but to my surprise I slowly began to improve. In a few years, I won National AAU titles at 25 and 30 kilometers and the RRC 50-miler. More important, I have enjoyed robust health and have been injury free for the eight years following my "enlightenment."

This article enunciates the guidelines I have evolved from this experience. I feel that these guidelines can produce good, predictable racing performances, while the runner maintains robust general health.

THE COMMON SENSE PRINCIPLE

And what is this revelation I claim? Is it some startling fact never previously observed? No indeed! How magnificent is nature in her understatement! I suffered for 10 years with injuries and erratic racing performance, only to find that nature herself has provided us with a simple common sense guide to determining when we are performing healthy work in contrast to self-abuse. It is simply this:

When we feel good, look good, and are alert and productive, our bodies will be adapting effectively to stresses (like running) which we place upon them. If we feel tired, pain, and are washed out, we need rest, not stress.

Simple common sense? Yes! But how many times have I heard runners and coaches say, "I felt tired in that race; I must need more work," or "A workout's no good unless it hurts," or "I did not try hard enough," etc.

The main general thrust of this article has been stated. Particulars follow to aid the runner in its everyday application.

DETECTING OVERSTRESS

If we train too little, we do not improve. If we overtrain, our bodies not only fail to improve, but injury and/or illness are likely induced. How can the runner decide upon the quantity of training which produces improvement?

I believe that a practical determination of this optimum quantity can be arrived at by first learning the symptoms of initial overstress. The optimum quantity of running is, then, the largest amount which *fails* to produce these symptoms. In practice, the amount varies from day to day, and the experienced runner learns to "feel in his bones" the appropriate training for that moment.

Here is a list of key symptoms:

Symptoms of Overstress

1. Mild leg soreness.
2. Lowered general resistance (evidenced by sniffles, headache, fever blisters, etc.).
3. Washed-out feeling and I-don't-care attitude.
4. Poor coordination (evidenced by general clumsiness, tripping, stubbing one's feet, poor auto driving, etc.).
5. Hangover from previous run.

I cannot overemphasize the importance of this list. If any of these symptoms is observed today, it is likely that yesterday's run was too hard to allow the body to adapt effectively to its stress and to improve. Instead of getting a little better, you've gotten a little worse. Easy running should now commence, and harder running be resumed *only* after all these symptoms disappear.

One should also note that all these symptoms are quite mild. They are not dramatic and are, unfortunately, all too often ignored because they seem trivial. But remember that when training effectively you should feel good.

The first symptom, mild leg soreness, is perhaps the most important. It means that the legs are too tired for any real work. It is in this fatigued state that the opportunity of injury becomes fertile. We might say that the legs are pregnant with injury. If the runner continues training hard for several days, so that this leg soreness remains, an injury will likely be born. If he rests or runs easily until the soreness disappears, injury will likely be aborted.

I believe that my discovery of this simple principle in 1964 has largely been responsible for the fact that I have not had even the slightest injury for the past eight years, in spite of the considerable quantity of long racing my legs endured.

Thus we see that the runner can best decide if workouts are too hard by observing their effects over the following 24 hours. Runners must avoid following a predetermined training schedule with ascetic zeal. A flexible mental attitude is required so that necessary corrections can be made. There is no surer way for a runner to drive himself into injury, illness and poor performance than to religiously follow a training schedule which is more than his body can effectively handle.

Athletes should also consider that continual overstress can produce problems from which they might never fully recover. Buddy Edelen's sciatic problems, Jim Peters' collapse in the 1954 Empire Games marathon, as well as problems endured by several lesser known runners I have observed, all marked the end of promising running careers. Symptoms of overstress must not be taken lightly.

HABITS WHICH HELP MINIMIZE OVERSTRESS

Besides recognizing the symptoms of overwork and stress, it is well to incorporate the following habits into the athlete's training program. These reduce the likelihood of overstress.

1. **Frequent easy days**—Some athletes train hard every other day, running easily on the remaining days. This makes good sense, as it tends to insure recovery.

2. **Flexible mental attitude**—There is no surer path to injury, poor health and bad racing than a stubborn dedication to a strict training schedule. No one can design in advance a training schedule which can anticipate the many variables the runner will encounter. Thus, "common sense" must always prevail, and a schedule must be abandoned or altered as the need arises.

3. **Good diet**—The runner's needs are not much different than those of the general public, except for perhaps increased fluid and caloric input. The runner should attempt to get his nourishment from *fresh natural* sources. Artificial food supplements, such as manufactured vitamins, are of dubious value.

4. **Wear good shoes**—A poor shoe is a sure source of injury. The shoe should have a *soft flexible* bottom to absorb road shock. The elevation of the heel is critical. This elevation should be identical on the runner's training and racing shoes, and at least as high as his dress shoes. If not, he will likely injure the tendons near his heel. The shoe must fit well, and must be kept in good repair. A great number of injuries are caused by worn shoes. In particular, the heel must be kept square at all times. As you train, the heels tend to wear on the outside. The runner must continually glue rubber to the worn area, or replace the heels. I replace the heels on my shoes about every 200 to to 250 miles.

5. **Quit races when exhausted**—Long distance races can be brutal on the runner's health. If the athlete runs too fast in the first few miles of a race, he should elect to retire rather than flog his body on while his nerves cry for relief. Every marathon race features a number of runners who make a point of seeing how much they can suffer. To be sure, they pay a high price in resultant injury and illness, for disregarding nature's warnings.

6. **Watch body weight**—A gain in weight of even a few pounds places a heavy additional strain on the runner. He should compensate by running slower, and adjusting his caloric input so as to return to his desired form.

RACING AND OVERSTRESS

While sprinting and running long distances at an easy speed are natural activities for man, racing long distances is not. One could appropriately describe participation in long distance racing as an act of *self-abuse*. Thus, the runner must consider carefully the frequency he will engage in this unnatural activity. He must also take special precautions to see that his body recovers from racing as quickly as possible.

Generally speaking, the longer the race, the longer will be the recovery period. The better the runner is conditioned, the sooner he will recover from a race of a given distance.

How often should one race? This is a complex question, which I try to answer in the following table. I assume that the runner is mature and is training about 75 miles per week.

1. Distance of Race	2. Minimum Recovery Period	3. Minimum Time Recommended Until Next Race	4. Special Notes
2 miles	24 hours	3 days	
5 miles	3 days	7 days	
10 miles	7 days	2 weeks	
15 miles	2 weeks	1 month	Not more than 5 15-milers recommended in a given year.
Marathon	1 month	3 months	Not more than two all-out marathons per year.
50 miles	3 months	1 year	Not more than one 50-miler every two years.

This table is only a general guide. Some athletes are naturally heartier than others, and can take more stress. Still others, better conditioned, will recover sooner. Nevertheless, I believe it realistically reflects the increase in stress caused by increasing racing distance, and the recovery periods required.

Meaning of the table:

Column 1: I assume that the runner goes "all-out" in this race.

Column 2: This minimum recovery period is the least time interval before the runner can repeat his performance. For example, if a runner clocks 54 minutes for 10 miles today, he can expect to repeat this performance in about one week. However, he could not continually race 10 miles each week without seriously risking damage to his health.

Column 3: While Column 2 gave the minimum recovery period, this column gives a realistic time interval after which the next race should take place. Thus, our 54-minute 10-miler, mentioned above, could expect to race 10 miles all-out every other week without risking eventual health damage.

Column 4: Races of 15 miles and more are sufficiently difficult that special precautions are necessary. These precautions are described.

My friends are likely to accuse me of hypocrisy, for I do race more often than I recommend in this table. *However, I do not race all-out.* For example, while I often race the marathon distance three, four or five times a year, only once, or perhaps twice, will I try to run as fast as I can. At other times I run considerably slower than I can on that day, so as to avoid abusing my health.

FINAL REMARK

As this article closes, it is well to repeat the "Common Sense Principle" stated in the first section: *You should look and feel good–be alert and productive when training effectively.* While many specific points were touched on such as shoe repair, racing frequency, etc., there is no substitute for your own analysis of your particular situation. Reflection on your own experiences, in the light of this basic Principle, should lead to a running career which not only provides satisfying racing performances, but robust health as well.

Chapter Two

Structural Problems

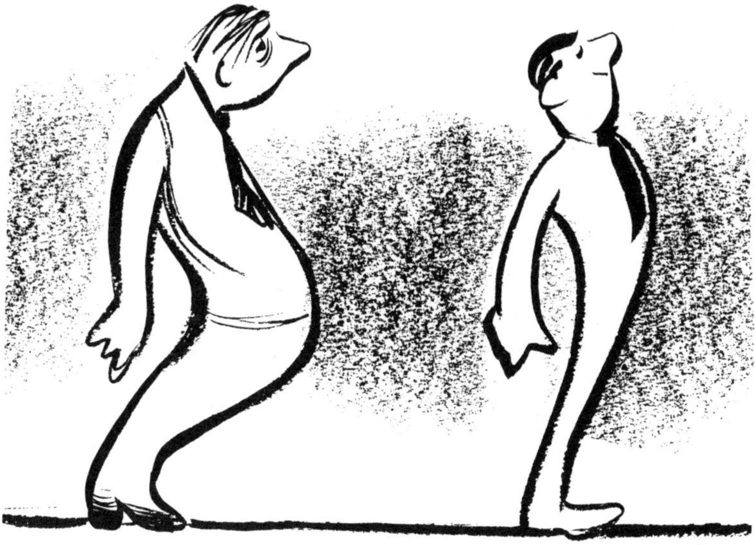

INTRODUCTION

Structural troubles—mainly those affecting the legs and their supporting tissues—give runners the most grief. Injuries vary with event. Hamstrings and bulky thigh muscles are the big target among sprinters. Distance men come down with knee and heel disabilities.

In 1971, Runner's World surveyed its reader-runners—almost all of them distance men. Eight hundred responded. The following percentages reported "structural" injuries serious enough to stop their running.

Knees	17.9%	Calves	3.6%
Achilles Tendons	14.0%	Heels	3.0%
Shin Splints	10.6%	Hips	2.6%
Arches	6.9%	Hamstrings	2.6%
Ankles	6.4%	Thighs	1.3%
Foot Fractures	4.9%	Leg Fractures	1.0%
Calves	3.6%		

The percentages are high, even though this study didn't take into account less serious but still aggravating injuries. They hobble nearly every runner at some time in his career.

Obviously, this booklet can't examine in detail every ailment that affects runners. That would encompass the entire field of medicine, which can't be condensed into a booklet this size. This chapter instead takes the most common problems of runners and focuses on them—again giving as much emphasis to prevention as to cure.

Muscle, bone, joint and tendon damage is primarily the result of two factors:

- Overuse (too much running, too fast).
- Inherent structural weakness.

The two actually work as one. Overuse makes the "weakest link" snap. Structural weaknesses, on the other hand, may cause one runner to snap at a level which is quite comfortable for another. To realize potential, one must know his limits.

Regardless of a runner's racing potential, he is only as strong as his structure. If the foundation isn't solid, nothing he has inside is going to do him much good.

FROM THE GROUND UP

BY GEORGE SHEEHAN, M.D.

The worst thing that ever happened to feet was shoes. Or perhaps the second worst, after concrete. These two products of urban civilization have finally conquered the human foot which in its primitive state crossed continents, pursued wild game and danced for days on end.

You may not think of the foot as man's crowning glory but it has been and is still capable of these incredible efforts. You may not think of the foot as reflecting the personality of its owner but it remains a key to the person's life style and state of health.

This is especially true of the athlete. His feet determine not only his physiological fitness but his instability as well. Unfortunately, the far-reaching effect of foot trouble on the rest of the body is not generally realized by the medical profession, or even by the podiatrists who make the diseases of the foot their specialty.

The foot bone, so the song goes, is connected to the ankle bone, and the ankle bone is connected to the leg bone, and the leg bone is connected to the thigh bone, and the thigh bone is connected to the hip bone, and the hip bone is connected to the back bone. So hear the word of the Lord. The foot bone is where we start to come apart.

The motto of sports physicians then should be, "Look to the athlete's feet regardless of his complaints."

There is Biblical evidence for such an approach. "The head cannot say to the feet, I have no need of thee!" says Paul in First Corinthians. "God has so adjusted the body that there may be no discord. If one member suffers all suffer together, if one member is honored all rejoice together."

Abraham Lincoln put it this way. "When my feet hurt, I can't think." Lincoln's blunt Anglo-Saxon makes more evident Paul's philosophic statement. It reaffirms the body-mind synthesis. And emphasizes, if it needs any emphasis, that man is his body.

It also tells us a universal truth. Painful feet affect saint and sinner, president and ward heeler, plodder and Olympian. And it reveals, since it implies a repeated event, that the Great Emancipator did more or less what we all do when we have trouble with our feet–nothing.

This resignation to the inevitable, this surrender to the belief that bad, weak and aching feet are just more evidence of man's frailty has carried over to the present day. I think it was Joan Crawford who asked, "Why is it when you say your foot hurts–it sounds all right, but when you say your *feet* hurt it sounds lousy?"

It sounds lousy because it contains the implication that your feet–and therefore all the rest of you–are made of bad material; that life, as you are living it, has proved you inadequate. And furthermore nothing can be done about it.

It is not true. The material is good. Shoes and concrete have done us in. That and transportation. "Civilized man," wrote Emerson, "has built a coach and lost the use of his feet," Brian Mitchell, a British national track coach, said recently that he could go through his entire working day and walk less than 100 yards. Over the centuries feet have always been able to adapt but not to inactivity.

But Lincoln's aching feet were the feet of an athlete. At 22 he weighed 180 pounds and was able, it was said, to outrun, outlift and outwrestle any man in Sangamon County, Ill. He once walked 34 miles one in day just to hear a famous lawyer argue a case in court. So Abe was no weekend athlete with a few blisters to show for over-activity. He was a counterpart of our present day athletes who are paying the cost of ignoring their feet.

"The feet are unquestionably the most abused and neglected part of the body," states Harvard trainer Jack Fadden. "They do the most work and receive the least attention. And the major reasons for foot problems, of course, are shoes." The greatest asset an athlete can have, according to Fadden, is a well fitted pair of shoes.

The conclusion, then, is good shoes or none at all. Walking barefoot on softer surfaces–sand and earth–is still the best of all foot exercises, and also lets us know that the foot is a major part of man's communication with his universe. The feel of sand, and dirt, and pine needles (what luxury!), the sensation of running in rain or over rocks, the immediacy and expression of all the surfaces can be felt through the feet.

If we must insert shoes between man and his environment, between man and his speech, let them be made to his imprint in the sand and to the sand's consistency.

"Man speaks with his whole body," wrote Sarte. "When he talks he speaks...when he runs he speaks..."

LOOK FIRST AT FEET

Most foot, leg, knee and hip troubles in runners are what the medical profession calls "overuse syndromes." Too many miles at too high speeds, according to this conventional wisdom, are the cause of stress fractures, shin splints, achilles tendonitis, knee pain, and innumerable other lesser known musculo-tendonous difficulties.

But evidence is accumulating that too-many-miles-too-fast is only part of the story. (Any number of perfectly healthy runners are handling the same distances/speeds.) Some biomechanical difficulty (malfunction in the running mechanism) has to be added to long mileage and high speed to cause disease. This biomechanical problem is most often in the foot.

- **Item**–Chondromalacia of the knee (a difficulty reported by almost 20% of *Runner's World* readers) of two years duration treated unsuccessfully with rest, cortisone shots, butazolidine. Cured by podiatrist's tailored foot inserts to correct arch problem.

• **Item**—College cross-country star with chondromalacia of knee and fluid in knee joint of three weeks duration cured with individualized support for pronated (unstable) foot with short first metatarsal (Morton's Foot). (For further discussion of chondromalacia, see page 47.)

• **Item**—Shin splints unresponsive to ultrasound, whirlpool. Cleared with molded crest under toes. Exercise of anti-gravity muscles added as preventive.

• **Item**—Achilles tendonitis remained symptomatic after cortisone injection and butazolidine. Helped with total foot support—anterior crest, wedged arch and heel lift.

• **Item**—Calf pull with 13 years of ineffectual medication and physiotherapy. Runner able to resume training after corrective inserts were made.

• **Item**—4:10 miler who lost entire freshmen year being treated for muscle pull just below back of knee. Got rid of pain when treated for pes cavus (very high arch).

• **Item**—Stress fracture of fibula apparently healed but with residual disabling pain. No help from medication. Runner free of symptoms after podiatrist made corrective insert for running shoes.

• **Item**— Heel spur problem. No success with doughnut heel support, cortisone shots. Relief of forefoot strain through corrective insert.

The foot is the primary cause of the majority of overuse syndromes, and a contributing cause to the remainder. When foot, ankle, knee problems start, you might try a Dr. Scholl's arch support. But should symptoms persist and inhibit running, a podiatrist (preferably with some interest in sports podiatry) should be consulted.

After 10 years of running at an age where, as Stan Musial once said, "You get hurt just standing around," I have experienced almost every conceivable overuse syndrome. In these instances, I must confess that my colleagues the orthopedic specialists have been of little use.

When I was helped in any way except by waiting it out, the podiatrist provided that help by fashioning or adjusting my foot supports. For muscle pulls, I found ultrasound gave good symptomatic therapy. Tendon pain seemed to be helped by whirlpool. The best and fastest help came from contrast baths—alternately cold and hot.

Muscle pulls of the thigh seem to be due to imbalance in muscular development. Where no hill work is done, the quadriceps are relatively weak and may pull. Gastrocnemius (calf) and hamstring pulls are unusual except in early training when they are still weak.

Low back pain is unusual, too, but sciatic pain (pain along the route of the sciatic nerve from sacroiliac joint and buttock down the back of the leg to the big toe) is almost always due to low-back problems. Chief of these is spondylolisthesis—a slippage of the spine on the pelvis—or excessive swayback.

Therapy is aimed toward straightening the back and rotating the pelvis forward. Sit-ups, sit-up curls, leg raises, buttock tightening and tummy-tucking

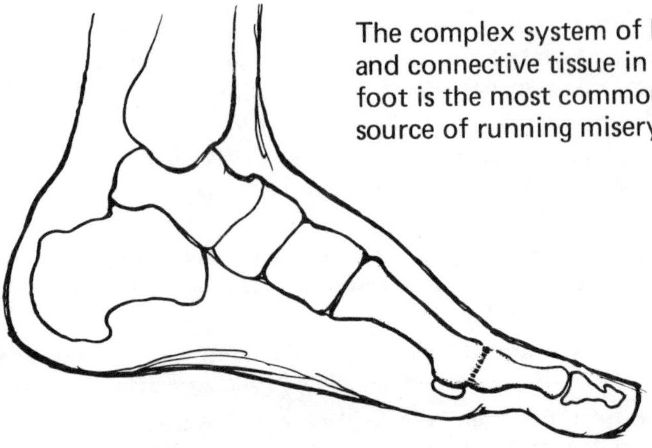

The complex system of bones and connective tissue in the foot is the most common source of running misery.

help. Flexibility exercises, especially for the hamstrings, are usually necessary. No-heel shoes, or barefoot walking should be encouraged. Use of a lumbosacral support has been reported to be quite helpful.

Summary: Overuse syndromes are due to mileage/pace plus a susceptible athlete. Cure lies not in reducing the effort or in getting symptomatic relief (i.e., cortisone, medicine, physiotherapy) but in finding the mechanical weakness—usually in the foot.

Otherwise, the athlete apparently cured by cortisone (heel spur and achilles), cast (stress fractures), rest (chondromalacia), physiotherapy (soleus and gastrocnemius pain) will have his symptoms return when he resumes running. *(BY GEORGE SHEEHAN, M.D.)*

IMBALANCE INJURIES

Is there anyone quite as forlorn as an injured athlete? Can you show me anyone as downcast as a sore-armed pitcher? Or as depressed as a fullback with a torn achilles? Do you know anyone as gloomy as an Olympian with a hamstring pull? Or a major leaguer with shin splints?

One would have to go back to blind Samson, or the deaf Beethoven, or the demented Nijinsky to glimpse what the loss of such perfection means. And despite the minor nature of these muscle problems, it is the loss of perfection we are talking about. Even though these injuries are often painless at rest and sometimes even in ordinary activity, they remove the athlete from his arena and what he does best.

It is easy to see why an ordinary American male with a scouting report of "good health, lousy shape" could pull one of his flabby muscles. But why a well-conditioned athlete at the peak of his training should suddenly come up with an incapacitating muscle or tendon injury continues to baffle the experts.

So this parade of game-legged runners files in and out of treatment rooms while nothing resembling a basic rule of prevention or treatment has been established by the medicos. No one has come up with a formula to prevent these catastrophes despite the fact that we are talking about athletes who command astronomical salaries or have world ranking in their events.

The reasons for this, I suspect, fall into two categories.

- The first is the assumption, common to all humanity, that someone else is working on the problem. Everyone, therefore, continues to use treatments long proved useless while they wait for the new information to come along.

- The second is that what thinking is being done is being done by paramedical personnel. These are people who do not have the standing in the scientific community to get their ideas spread around and accepted. They don't have the authority, real or imagined, that an M.D. commands.

But in the *New York Times* sports section one of these men, a physiotherapist named Joseph Zohar, found a forum for a new program to "reduce injuries, prevent muscle strains and probably improve the performance of the athletes using it." (See page 53 for further details.)

It is Zohar's theory that the athlete needs preventive exercises rather than conditioning exercises. "Conditioning a pitcher's arm through pitching alone," he states, "does not provide a high degree of protection against muscle strains and injuries." Such protection comes only when the athlete has each muscle in the arm individually exercised. "Even one poorly conditioned muscle" Zohar writes, "can make the arm vulnerable."

So he recommends that each muscle group be exercised to improve strength, endurance and range of motion. This insures that no weakness, tightness or insufficient endurance of a single muscle is left uncorrected. The basic idea is that all muscle pulls are due to imbalance in strength, endurance or flexibility.

I tend to agree. Some time ago, I looked into this problem and was struck by the relative immunity of basketball players to the muscle ailments of other athletes. Muscle pulls are almost non-existent. Even though basketball players accelerate and charge down the court at top speed on fast breaks, change pace dramatically and are forever leaping around under the backboard, nothing seems to happen to them.

When other athletes, however, are exposed to basketball, the result is carnage. Ask a track coach about basketball and he mourns over his injured runners. Achilles tears, calf pulls and thigh strains are common occurrences when stars of other sports move into basketball.

So the lack of muscle pulls and strains among basketball players is not due to the game itself. It is as demanding physically as any other sport. Perhaps even more so. Yet in some way it prevents its own players from getting into trouble.

The answer, it seems to me, must be the same as Zohar's plan for the pitchers. Basketball exercises every muscle in the leg. Most sports are straight ahead on the flat. Most sports demand strength or endurance, not both. But basketball is all-demanding. Speed plus strength plus endurance plus flexibility is required in this ballet of sports. The basketball player must develop the muscles that lift the leg (the antigravity muscles) as well as those that push it off. Running backwards, a quite ordinary activity for a basketball player, will uncover muscles a long distance runner never knew he had.

That is the remarkable thing. A runner who puts in 50 or 60 miles a week can find muscles in his legs he is apparently not even using, or at least not using to the extent that their capacity for strength, endurance and flexibility is anywhere near developed. It makes Zohar's theory believable.

Zohar is simply recommending the preventive exercises used in the field of rehabilitation. Furthermore, he says, such programs would consume only a fraction of the time spent daily on training.

It may seem too good to be true, but this looks like the answer to those old muscle-pulling, shin-splinting, heel-cord-ripping, whatever-happened-to-my-hamstring blues. *(BY GEORGE SHEEHAN, M.D.)*

STRESSES AND STRAINS

BY WILLIAM CLANCY, M.D.

Dr. Clancy, a former distance runner, is chief resident in the Department of Orthopedic Surgery at St. Luke's Hospital Center, New York City. St. Luke's houses a sports medicine clinic, which Clancy founded.

In this article, I will explain and define the most common injuries among runners: (1) strains, (2) sprains, (3) stress fractures, (4) tendonitis.

STRAIN— *a tear in the muscle-tendon complex.* It is graded "first-degree" if minimal to mild, "second-degree" if moderate, and "third-degree" if complete.

Unless this complex is completely torn, there is no accurate way to tell how severe the tear is. The amount of pain, swelling and muscle spasm help make the classification as to first- or second-degree. This classification is significant because a first-degree injury should heal readily and allow early return to full training. However, a second-degree is a significant injury and requires careful and cautious treatment; otherwise too early return to running may cause delay in healing, thus more scar formation. This in turn will result in more pain, less pliability of the joint and a longer rehabilitation period before full training can be resumed. The greatest danger is that of converting a second- to a third-degree (complete rupture) occasionally seen in achilles tendonitis.

Athletes who have sustained a second- or third-degree strain will have healed with significant amount of scar tissue. Muscle fibers do not regenerate, thus do not heal muscle fiber to muscle fiber. Rather, the gap is bridged by scar tissue which lacks the properties of muscle—namely elasticity and tone. Before returning to full training after such an injury, an athlete must do stretching and strengthening exercises; otherwise he risks injury or constant pain during running.

SPRAIN—*a tear in a ligament.* Ligaments are strong fibrous bands that hold joints together. They likewise are classified as first-, second- or third-degree sprains. Not all third-degree sprains need surgery, but they do need some form of complete immobilization.

In runners, the most common sprain is a first- or second-degree sprain of their lateral ligaments of the ankle. A first-degree sprain should be treated initially with ice and elevation for 24 to 48 hours, followed by a two- to three-day rest.

A second-degree sprain requires the same initial treatment, but the resting period may require up to six weeks, depending on the number of ligaments torn. Pain to pressure over the ligaments is generally a very good guide as to when one can resume training. One should not even start straight ahead jogging if there is any pain to pressure.

STRESS FRACTURES— *bone damage.* In the past year and a half, we have seen 15 stress fractures in high school and college runners. Contrary to the classical "march fracture" (metetarsal fracture) most of ours have been in the tibia or fibula of the lower leg.

They often appear to be severe "shin splints" and could very easily be misdiagnosed. A fracture line generally does not appear on an x-ray until symptoms have been present for approximately two to three weeks, and sometimes even four weeks. Generally, these fractures do not need cast immobilization (depending on the fracture and its location). One cannot begin training until there is good x-ray evidence of complete bony union; otherwise one is inviting disaster.

TENDONITIS– *tendon inflammation.* This and chondromalcia of the patella are the two greatest injuries seen in our clinic, and probably everywhere. Tendonitis is an inflammation of the tubular sheath surrounding a tendon. In runners, the most commonly affected tendon is the achilles.

In my opinion, there are two different mechanisms of injury. The first and least common is that of direct and constant pressure on the tendon sheath. This was common during World War II from the combat boot. It is also occassionally seen after too tight an ankle strapping with non-elastic tape. A very high counter (back support) on a shoe may also cause this.

The most common cause, in my opinion, is a stress tear of the tendon. Once there is a partial tear, and this is probably a microscopic tear, it will start to heal itself. Since tendon has no blood supply of its own, it must receive it from somewhere else. The blood supply is from the tendon sheath. Therefore, the sheath becomes secondarily inflamed. It becomes thickened, and since it is tubular the inner diameter becomes smaller.

The tendon cannot glide up and down this tube now without a great deal of friction. If it does so, it will continue this inflammatory reaction which initially started to heal the partial tendon tear. The tear will heal, but the inflammatory process will continue because of the constant friction. Until the inflammatory reaction has been allowed to resolve, friction will be present and the inflammation will be perpetuated. It is mandatory that rest be taken to allow the inflammation to subside. Anti-inflammatory agents and ice are quite beneficial at this stage.

I feel that steroids (cortisone) are not recommended at the initial reaction because the initial inflammatory reaction is necessary to heal the partial tendon tear. Proper initial recognition and treatment is mandatory; otherwise the likelihood of chronic achilles tendonitis is ever present.

After an acute injury, the injured part should be rested from activity. Ice should be applied four to five times for approximately 20 minutes during the first 24 to 48 hours. Rest, elevation and ice will act to diminish the initial swelling. Although the size of the swelling is not necessarily directly related to the severity of the injury, the greater the swelling, the longer the healing will take.

After the first 48 hours, certain techniques may be utilized to promote healing:

- Whirlpool can be used best for extremity strains or sprains. The object is to apply heat to the area of injury only. The blood vessels in the injured and surrounding area are thus selectively dilated, aiding the healing process. Whirlpool also combines heat with a gentle massaging action, further increasing blood flow to the injured area. If heat is applied to too great an area, there will be less blood flow to the injured area.

- To utilize a whirlpool four times a day for 20 minutes is generally not possible. A hydrocollator pack applied to the specific area will probably be just as efficient and more practical.

- Other substitutes would be a hot water bottle, a heating pad, or even hot towels.

- There are other heat modelities, but they have limitations. Ultrasound is best utilized in very small areas, about the size of a quarter.

- Diathermy has its best results in those with paraspinal muscle spasm. This can cause severe burns and should be used only by those who are qualified to do so.

- Infrared also has a very limited use and can likewise cause severe burns.

- Contrast soaks, that is the use of alternating hot and cold applications, is presently being utilized more and more. It appears to have promising results when used by the teenager and young adult. The older athlete—40s, 50s and 60s—does not appear to obtain the same improvements with it.

One must not forget, however, that initial resting of the injured part is by far the most important part of any rehabilitation program and the above are only aids to the entire healing process.

TREATING WITH WATER

"Cool it!" This appears to be the best possible advice when soft-tissue injuries (primarily to the muscles and tendons) happen.

Immediate cool-it treatment involves (1) a modification of running—amount determined by the severity of the injury, and (2) application of just plain cold water.

Animals in the wilds have been observed using this method when they get hurt. Deer, which must keep running to eat and survive, stand in streams to cool their aching legs.

Soft-tissue injuries are accompanied by inflammation. The symptoms of inflammation are redness, heat, swelling, pain and limitation of movement. When the deer feels heat in his injured leg, instinct leads him to the cold stream.

Athletic medicine has taken the lesson of the deer and is applying the same principle—cooling injured muscles and tendons with either cold water or ice.

The first 48 hours after the injury occurs is considered the crucial period. Immediate and repeated cold applications reduce inflammation, which in turn slows swelling. Heat, in any form, during this first two-day period should be avoided since it has just the opposite, undesirable effect.

Common methods of applying cold are hanging the injured part under a running tap, soaking it in a pan or bucket, rubbing with ice cubes, or packing in ice (wrapping in an ice-filled stocking is one way).

After the first crucial two-day period, water-treatment is still generally advised. But the *type* of water used is the subject of some controversy.

Conventional medical opinion is the water should be hot. The reasoning behind this is that hot water breaks up the waste products that have collected around the injury.

However, success has been reported recently with the continuous application of cold until the pain has vanished—or at least alternating cold and hot treatment. The reason continued cold may be beneficial, even after the first two days, is this: the runner is one of the few patients who reinjures himself daily. Each workout may cause damage, though so slight it's almost unnoticed. Applying cold after each run may keep this new damage in check while healing progresses.

The American Medical Association cautions, however, that continuous cold "should be regarded as an experimental method of therapy until fully documented reports of investigations on this approach are available for study."

References: *Denis Wright, Athletics Weekly, July 25, 1970; Leonard Hibbert, Athletics Weekly, Aug. 15, 1970; Fred Hein, Sports and Physical Fitness/JAMA Questions and Answers; Joe Henderson, Runner's World, May 1972.*

THE COMPLEX ARCHES

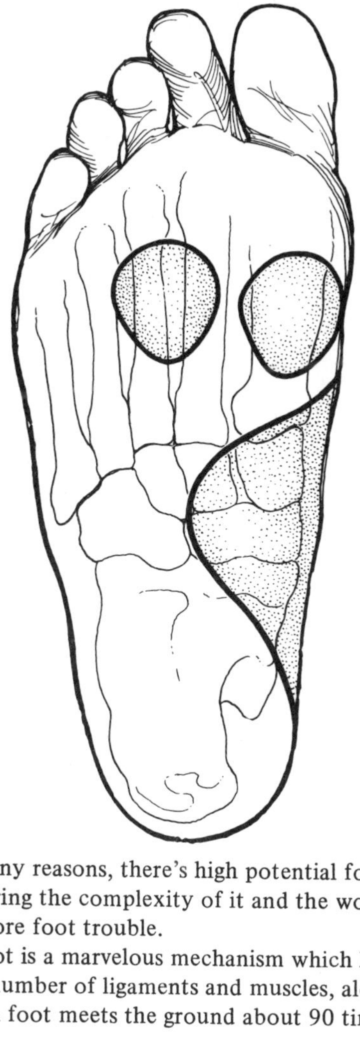

Metatarsal pads (above) and longitudinal arch support (below) are two of the corrective devices for foot problems.

For many reasons, there's high potential for trouble in the foot. In fact, considering the complexity of it and the work it bears, it's surprising there isn't more foot trouble.

The foot is a marvelous mechanism which has 26 bones, and almost double that number of ligaments and muscles, along with a few bursa. While running, each foot meets the ground about 90 times a minute—or 5000 times an hour.

According to a survey made by a British governmental agency in 1966, six out of every 10 people have basic abnormalities of their feet. Perhaps the best way to tell what is abnormal in feet is to first list the characteristics of *normal* ones.

- **The foot is free of pain.**
- **The heel is centrally located under the leg.**
- **The toes are straight and flexible.**
- **The muscular control is well-balanced.**

- **The foot is flexible, with no soft-tissue contractures.**
- **The heel-toe motion is proper during gait.**

Apparently, over half of us lack one or more of these characteristics. So what happens? When the basically weak foot pounds the ground several thousand times a day, an injury is likely to result. Even normal stresses on such abnormal feet may cause pain—not only in the foot itself, but in the achilles tendon, calf, shins, knees and other areas as well.

The most common abnormalities of the feet center on one of the three arches:

1. *Longitudinal inner arch*—along the inside of the foot, extending from just in front of the heel to the base of the first long toe joint.

2. *Lateral longitudinal arch*—in the same position on the outside of the foot.

3. *Metatarsal arch*—across the ball of the foot.

They may be too high or too flat to begin with, or they may fall when stressed. If one of the arches falls, several things can happen. One is that a long tendon running up the leg (the posterior tibial tendon) is stretched. Pain develops high in the calf and gravitates down toward the ankle. Eventually the pain reaches the arch proper and the plantar fascia (the sheet of tissue across the bottom of the foot).

Also, falling arches can result in a turning in or "pronating" of the foot to compensate. This leads to an unnatural footfall, with increased possibilities of injury to the feet and legs.

The best long-range treatment for all foot abnormalities—innate and acquired—appears to be the use of corrective inserts. These, in effect, put the foot back in natural balance.

References: *Rene Cailliet, AFP/GP, November 1970; George Sheehan, All About Distance Running Shoes, July 1971; George Sheehan, Runner's World, September 1971.*

CARING FOR BLISTERS

Blisters are every runner's companion. Regardless of the improvements in shoes and protective measures taken, foot blisters continue to be a fact of life in running. But they are a major problem only (1) when they are severe enough to affect running quantity, quality or technique; (2) when infection develops.

Foot blisters are caused by heat; they are essentially burns produced by friction. The best way to prevent blisters is to prevent the friction that causes them. Here are several recommendations:

1. Buy high-quality shoes (without improperly-placed stitching, rough edges, etc.) and be sure they fit comfortably.

2. Take care of the shoes. Don't let the uppers get so brittle or the insoles so worn that "hot-spots" might develop.

3. Never wear new shoes in a race (or even in a long workout where there'll be no opportunity to change). Each pair of shoes breaks in the feet, as well as being broken in itself. The shoes and the feet must become accustomed to each other.

What about socks? This is the source of some controversy. Opinion is split between those who say wearing socks *prevents* blisters, and those who say socks *cause* them. This much is clear: Modern running shoes don't require layers of sock for protection between them and the feet. And with socks, you run the risk of irritating folds developing as you go along. If you wear socks, wear clean, snug-fitting ones.

When blisters do bubble up, the goals of treatment are to keep yourself running without impairment and to prevent infection. These can be accomplished by:

- Keeping the area clean—especially if the blister has broken.

- *Not* puncturing small blisters immediately.

- Puncturing blisters that cause pressure and pain. Puncture the clean blister with a sterile needle to release fluid, squeezing gently with a sterile gauze. *Do not remove the skin.*

- Padding (with gauze and possibly foam rubber) and taping open blisters.

- Continuing to run if you can do so without significant pain and alteration of running form.

- Consulting a physician or podiatrist at the first sign of infection or complication.

Reference: *Bob Carman, Guide to Distance Running.*

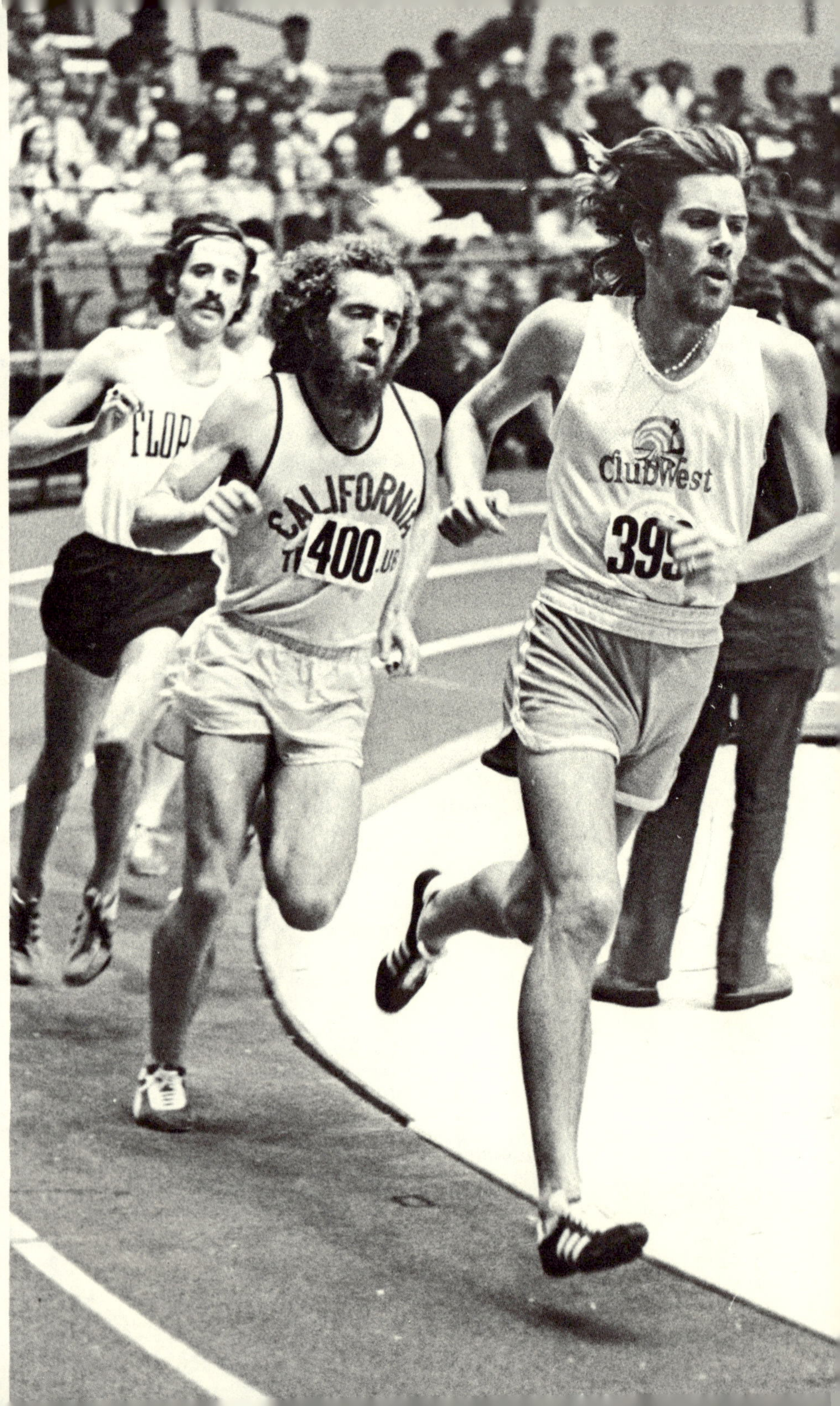
FLOR
CALIFORNIA
400
ClubWest
399

ACHILLES TENDONS

Three words of advice apply to the achilles tendons more than anywhere else. *Don't hurt them!*

Achilles tendon injuries are miserable. They not only disrupt running, but they keep disrupting it for a long, long time. In fact, there's considerable evidence to support the statement: "Once an achilles victim, always an achilles victim." Once you injure this sensitive tendon that connects the calf and the heel bone, you're susceptible to reinjury with increasingly less provocation. Unless you watch your step and modify or eliminate basic causes, you will surely be out of action again sooner or later.

Heel injuries rank with knee damage as the most prevalent and discouraging ailments in running. They're quick to strike and slow to heal–if they ever truly heal.

British sports medicine expert Denis Wright has written extensively on the achilles. He identifies three main types (or degrees) of damage:

- **Tendonitis**–an inflammation of the tendon.
- **Partial rupture**–tearing of the tendon fibers.
- **Complete rupture**–complete break in the tendon.

Each is more serious (and less common) than the one before. Let's look at them one at a time.

TENDONITIS

Causes: (a) a sudden change in routine (e.g., a change in footwear–flats to spikes; a change in surface–grass to cinders; a change in training–endurance to speed); (b) by ignoring the reaction to a heavy training session or race.

Symptoms: (a) awareness of pain and stiffness an hour or so following activity, particularly after rest; (b) slight swelling, often only detectable by the experienced eye; (c) pain on contraction and stretching of calf muscles; (d) tenderness to squeezing pressure applied at the tendon's narrowest point; (e) walking possible, running difficult, sprinting impossible.

PARTIAL RUPTURE

Causes: (a) a weakness due to long-standing tendonitis; (b) a sudden stretching applied while the calf muscles are contracting vigorously.

Symptoms: (a) a history of tendonitis; (b) onset of pain sudden and during activity; (c) obvious swelling, apparent within an hour; (d) pain on contraction, much more severe on stretch; (e) hypersensitivity to squeezing pressure; (f) walking is difficult; running, other than the slowest jog, is impossible.

Page 38: The combination of high speeds and tight cornering creates problems for indoor runners. (Don Chadez photo)

COMPLETE RUPTURE

Causes: (a) a direct blow to a tense tendon; (b) a logical sequence following tendonitis and partial rupture; (c) those likely to cause a partial rupture.

Symptoms: the heel is detached from the calf muscle, leaving the leg useless; an extremely serious injury requiring immediate surgery.

For our purposes here, we only need to talk about the first two types—except to mention that ignoring the first two can lead to complete rupture. Any runner who reaches this point isn't going to be able to think about running again until he has had surgery and a long period of rehabilitation—if then.

Diagnosis and treatment begin the instant achilles tendon damage is detected. Read your pains. If you are walking with a slight limp, you probably have tendonitis. If you have a severe limp but can still hobble around, you may have a more serious partial rupture—a tear in the tendon.

Immediate self-treatment for these injuries can be summarized in one sentence: *If it hurts, cool it.* This has two meanings:

1. *Apply cold water or ice to the injured area* (see article on water treatment in this chapter).

2. *Use pain as a guide.* Reduce activity to the point where it isn't intolerably painful. Slow down or stop if pain grows worse while exercising. If you aren't hurting, you probably aren't hurting yourself.

In the early stages of an achilles injury, stretching should be avoided. Overstretching led to the problem. While pain is acute, don't tempt fate by stretching the tendon even more. Wear well-heeled shoes. Run on smooth, flat and straight surfaces. Stay away from speedwork.

In most cases, it is possible to continue running at reduced distances and paces while the tendon is healing. Don't expect all traces of the injury to vanish quickly. These are among the slowest healing of injuries.

As long as there is apparent inflammation and acute pain, applications of ice or cold water after each running session may prove valuable. However, this is merely the treatment of symptoms. Eventually you have to give some thought to eliminating basic causes, which in turn will reduce chances of chronic, recurring injuries in the weakened tendon.

Step One in the long-range prevention plan is to induce stretching. This is the opposite of the suggestion for immediate treatment. A cause of tendon injuries appears to be their shortness and inflexibility. This partly results from the fact that we always wear shoes with substantial heels. When the runner stretches out for speed, the tendon can't handle the unaccustomed stretch. It rebels.

Suggested stretching exercises for the achilles tendon include (1) leaning into the wall for modified pushups, and (2) standing with the balls of the feet on a step and bouncing gently so the heels go lower than the toes.

Another worthwhile stretching procedure appears to be the gradual lowering of heels on both running shoes and street shoes, and walking barefoot whenever possible.

Step Two in prevention is to avoid sudden and violent changes in routine. Go gradually from slow work to fast, from the flats to the hills, from the track to the road, from low mileage to high.

Step Three relates to the first two. Watch what you put on your feet. Shoes control tendon stretching. You must reach a happy medium where the tendon stretches enough but not too much. So it's imperative that you find a shoe that does this and then stick with it. Race and train in the same shoe if possible. And at the very least don't make sudden, drastic shifts in heel height.

The suggestions here apply to achilles victims and potential victims alike. Everyone who runs is either on or the other.

References: *Denis Wright, Athletics Weekly, July 25, 1970; Joe Henderson, Runner's World, May 1972.*

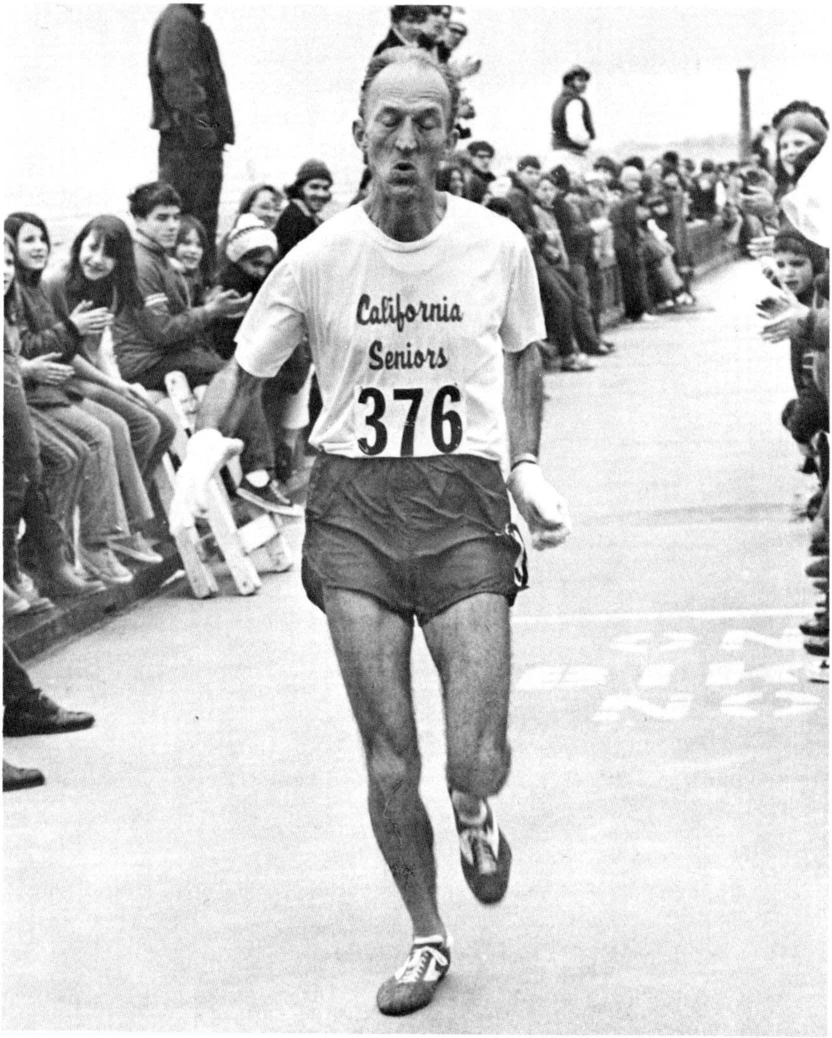

Road men have the highest incidence of achilles trouble. (Herriott)

HEEL BONE DAMAGE

Runners shouldn't get the impression that all heel injuries—in fact, all injuries *period*—can be treated simply by modifying activity and/or splashing on a little cold water. Some progress to where there's no avoiding major medical care. The heels are peculiarly susceptible to this kind of damage.

A prime target is the spot where the heel bone and the achilles tendon meet. Irritation at this point—poorly made shoes have gotten part of the blame—can cause one or two things to occur.

- The bursa (protective sacs around the heel and tendon) become inflammed and quite painful.

- Continued irritation leads to the development of bony growth on the point of the heel, which in turn can cut into the achilles tendon and cause a chronic partial rupture.

A doctor may need to inject cortisone into the troublesome bursa, or in advanced cases may have to remove the sac altogether.

In the case of bony growth that damages the tendon, surgery is required. The doctor has to cut into the heel and scrape away the calcium deposit so the tendon will again have a smooth groove in which to slide. If tendon damage is advanced, the surgery may also include repair of the achilles.

Many runners also develop painful "spurs" on the bottoms of their heels—at the point where the heel bone connects with the plantar fascia. Some relief can be had by using a "donut-style" pad in that area. A good arch support may help by relieving pressure on the plantar fascia. As a last resort, surgery is sometimes necessary.

References: *Arthur Lydiard, Runner's World, July 1970; Bob Carman, Runner's World, November 1970; Joe Henderson, Runner's World, May 1972.*

LEG AND FOOT BURSITIS

Potentially painful bursa are the closed sacs which protect areas subject to friction. They are filled with fluid. When friction at one of these contact points—such as the area where a tendon passes over a bone—is unusually heavy, painful bursitis can develop.

Bursitis can occur in one of several locations:

- Under the kneecap.
- Between the groin muscle and the hip.
- On the bony prominence of thigh just below the hip.
- Between achilles tendon and heel bone.
- In the big toe.

Medical relief may be obtained one of two ways if the case is severe: (1) through drugs (butazolidine, or injection of cortisone); (2) surgery to remove the bursa.

Reference: *Arthur Lydiard, Runner's World, July 1970.*

SHIN SPLINT CAUSES

Shin splints are pains, usually with swelling, along the front of the lower leg. Although shin splints are primarily a muscular problem, they have many of the same symptoms as stress fractures which occur in the same area.

Many researchers have concluded that shin splints are transmitted from a faulty foot plant.

According to Australian sports physician A. B. Corrigan, they are due to the "controlled elongation" of the muscle as the foot drives off the ground. Restricting the driving motion of the toes with a rubber toe crest can help.

Inflexible shoes have also been identified as a potential culprit. When the sole of the shoe hits the ground and refuses to bend, unusual shock is produced. This shock may be absorbed—to a greater degree than normal—by the shin muscles (anterior tibial).

In another study related to running form, William F. Leach of the University of Illinois/Chicago Circle, concluded that the angle at which the foot hits the ground is the crucial factor. The study included four runners with chronic shin splint problems and three who had never had them.

Leach filmed the runners in action. He discovered that the feet and legs of the non-sufferers were straighter (more in line with hip and knee) on landing than those of the victims. The "angles of adduction" were 7.67 degrees in the right leg for the healthy runners, compared to 9.75 degrees for the men with shin splints. In the left leg, the figures were 10.0 and 15.75 degrees. The greater angle put greater stress on the shin, the researcher said, and "repeated velocity, or over an extended period of time, could possibly result in musculo-tendonous strain."

Also, an imbalance between the weak anterior tibial muscle and a strong calf muscle may be a factor. The treatment would be muscle development of the front of the leg.

References: *Medical Tribune, Aug. 25, 1971; A. B. Corrigan, Medical Journal of Australia, July 22, 1967.*

ANTERIOR UPPER LEG

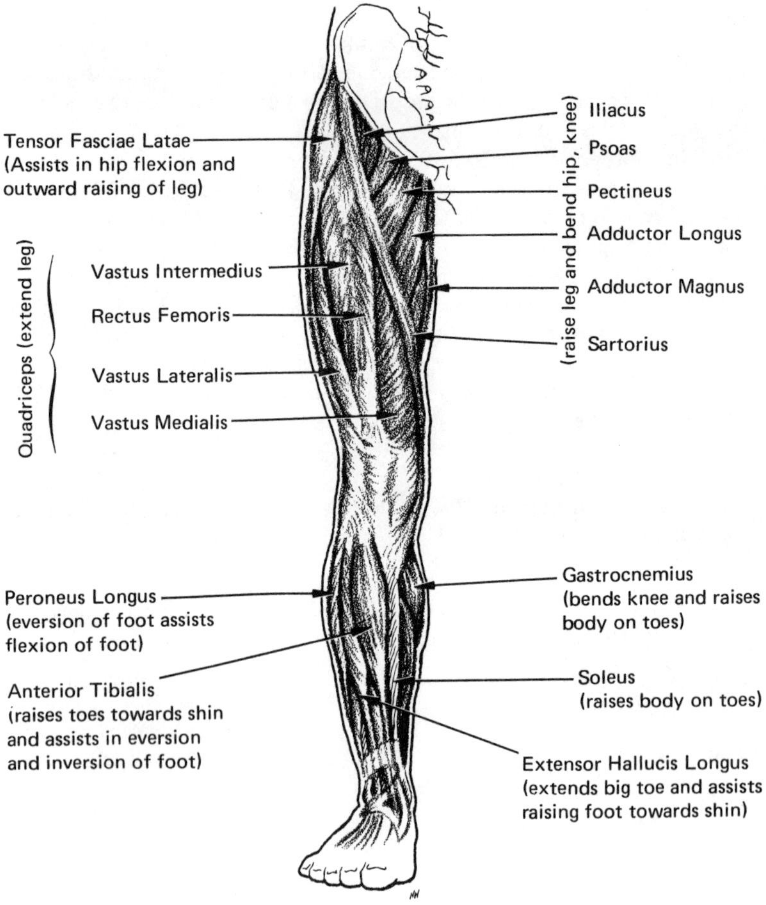

Reprinted from "Strength, Power and Muscular Endurance" by John Jesse

POSTERIOR UPPER LEG

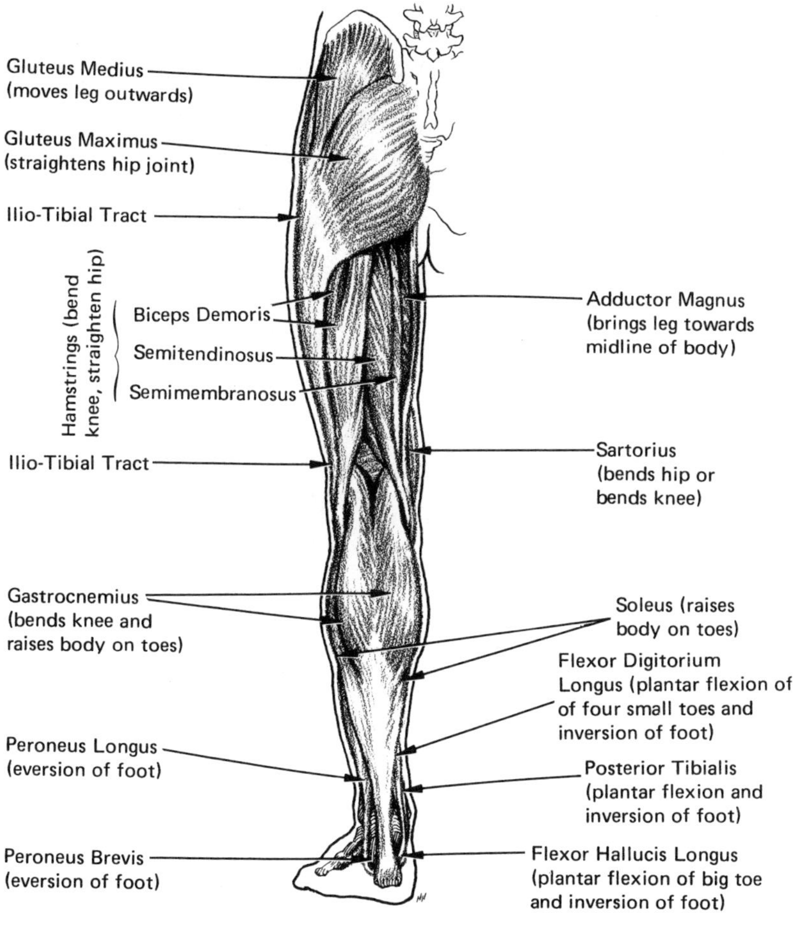

Reprinted from "Strength, Power and Muscular Endurance" by John Jesse

STRESS FRACTURES

We tend to associate the word "fracture" with traumatic events. Stress fractures aren't that way. They come on so subtly, in most cases, that most athletes–and even some doctors– may mistake them for "shin splints" or "foot bruises."

Dr. Frederick Behling, team physician at Stanford University, showed why this mistake is made when he spelled out the symptoms of stress fracture. They strongly resemble those of shin splints and deep bruises.

"The classic history in the athlete (with a stress fracture)," said Behling, "is one of vague but persistent pain in the lower extremity...in a performer subjecting himself to volume workouts where there has been a recent increase in volume. Running on hard surfaces is (also) thought to be an important factor."

Stress fractures, Behling said, have the following characteristics:

- General involvement of the shaft of a long bone.
- Onset without violence.
- Frequent association with prolonged muscle effort.
- Absence of an audible "snap."
- Absence of any suspicion by the patient that a fracture has occurred.

Over a period of 10 years, Behling treated 30 cases of stress fractures (about half in the foot, half in the lower leg). Twenty-three of the victims were runners–and all but two of them middle or long distance men.

"Track and cross-country athletes are by far the most frequent victims of stress fractures," Behling said. "In seven of the cases reviewed, the athletes sustained second fractures–three involving the same bone, and four involving different bones. All of these (repeated) injuries were sustained by middle or long distance runners."

Treatment for stress fractures usually involves a limitation of activity. Complete rest or immobilization are seldom required, Dr. Behling indicated, though he said exercise should be "reduced within the limits of comfort." Stress fractures normally mend within six weeks.

The cases of repeated injury among Stanford runners, however, hint that simply healing the fracture is not enough. Resumption of running without investigating basic mechanical problems in the feet and shoes, and without recognizing signs and symptoms of stress may lead to recurrence.

References: *Medical Tribune, April 21, 1969; Richard Elton, Journal of the American Medical Association, April 22, 1968.*

KNEE CHONDROMALACIA

BY GEORGE SHEEHAN, M.D.

Chondomalacia of the patella (knee cap) is one of the most frequently encountered athletic injuries. Almost 20% of distance runners polled by *Runner's World* had suffered knee symptoms sufficient to interrupt and even end their running careers. Also America's new middle-aged athletes, according to reports of the American Academy of Orthopedic Surgeons, are limping to physicians in record numbers with knee problems. The majority have chondromalacia.

Yet the origins of this disease remain a mystery. Recent reviews on the subject confirm a lack of consensus on what initiates and continues the damage on the patella. The literature also reveals a variety of recommended therapies. Rest leads the way, followed by butazolidine steroid injections, immobilization, quadricep exercises, and a variety of operations. None of these seems to afford more than temporary relief.

Recently, my personal experience as a runner, along with that of a veteran long distance man, has convinced me that chondromalacia in many, if not most, instances stems from an imbalance in the foot.

I first noted in my daily run that traveling against traffic was a painless outing. But should I run with traffic, I would soon develop pain in my left knee, which would worsen with each outing. The apparent cause of this knee difficulty was that the crown of the road caused me to run on the inside of my left foot traveling with traffic, but on the outside while going against it.

Shortly thereafter, I began corresponding with a first-class runner who had been suffering with typical chondromalacia symptoms for more than two years. Running with severe pain, he was able to confirm the fact that running on the outside of the foot relieved his symptoms.

Unfortunately, we did not make the next logical step until he developed arch symptoms. He then had inserts made and soon was running long distances without trouble. Within a short time, he ran the fastest marathon of his career.

His case and two others are briefly summarized:

- **Case One**: T.B., 26-year-old ex-Marine with two-year history of chondromalacia; treated with rest, butazolidine, steroid injections. Free of pain after molding and casting of foot supports by his podiatrist.

- **Case Two**: G.J., 23-year-old distance runner with two months of knee pain, worse while running and after inactivity; diagnosed as chondromalacia. Seen by podiatrist and found to have short first metatarsal with foot imbalance. After insertion of corrective support, became free of symptoms. In 10 days returned to number one position on his team.

- **Case Three**: 28-year-old with three-month history of knee pain due to chondomalacia; unimproved by rest. On his own bought arch supports, placed them in shoes, and "in one week I was able to run with no pain whatsoever."

Chondromalacia is an overuse syndrome of unknown causes. Evidence is presented here that the additional factor of overuse (which in the case of a runner is 90 foot strikes a minute for an hour a day) is a peculiarly susceptible individual. That susceptibility arises from an unstable foot with some mechanical imbalance transmitted to the knee and causing the patella to override on the lateral condyle (groove).

Runners find relief from: (A) Running so the crown throws the runner on the outside of the foot; (B) Reversing direction on the track to do the same thing; (C) Using corrective inserts. Success with these treatments confirms the foot as the origin of this pathology.

Overuse alone is not the cause. Many athletes are completely symptom-free while doing 70-100 miles a week, or more, while others develop pain on a much lighter program.

We need a fresh look at all overuse syndromes of the leg, knee, hip and back to see if abnormalities of the foot are responsible in these instances. The fact that some runners have repeated stress fractures (I know of one runner who had a stress fracture every year in college) points to some basic mechanical problem involving the foot and leg relationship.

This basic difficulty must be diagnosed before we can give overuse victims anything more than palliative treatment. Our best help in these diseases is a thorough investigation of the foot and the foot strike. Podiatrists, who give invaluable diagnosis and practical treatment along with molding and casting of corrective inserts, should be consulted.

"RUNNER'S KNEE" SYMPTOMS

BY WILLIAM CLANCY, M.D.

The most common problem for track athletes in our athletic clinic (as with athletes questioned by *Runner's World*) is chondromalacia of the patella. This means that the joint cartilage of the kneecap has been, or is being, destroyed.

This problem is caused by numerous anatomical variations in the knee joint. The patella is a V-shaped bone which glides over the femoral condyles, which are U-shaped. For numerous reasons, the patella may not be centered directly, but instead rides more on the lateral condyle. This causes increased friction and wear, and then destruction of the cartilage of the patella. What you have, then, is similar to what happens when a car wheel is out of alignment and the tire shows abnormal tread wear.

Several self-tests may indicate whether you have chondromalacia:

1. Is your pain directly under your kneecap?
2. Is your knee stiff in the morning?
3. Do you have pain climbing stairs (and if so is it under your kneecap)?
4. Do you have pain in your knees after prolonged sitting?
5. Do you ever have the feeling that your kneecaps are slipping out when running downhill or uphill?

6. Has your knee ever swollen up?

7. Have you ever had your knee lock on you where you were unable to flex it or extend it?

8. Has your knee ever given way?

9. If you lie on your back, flex your hips to 90 degrees and then flex your knees fairly rapidly all the way, do you feel grinding beneath your knee-caps?

10. If you lie flat on your back with your knees straight, and someone holds your kneecaps while you make the muscles in your thighs tight, do you get marked pain in your knees?

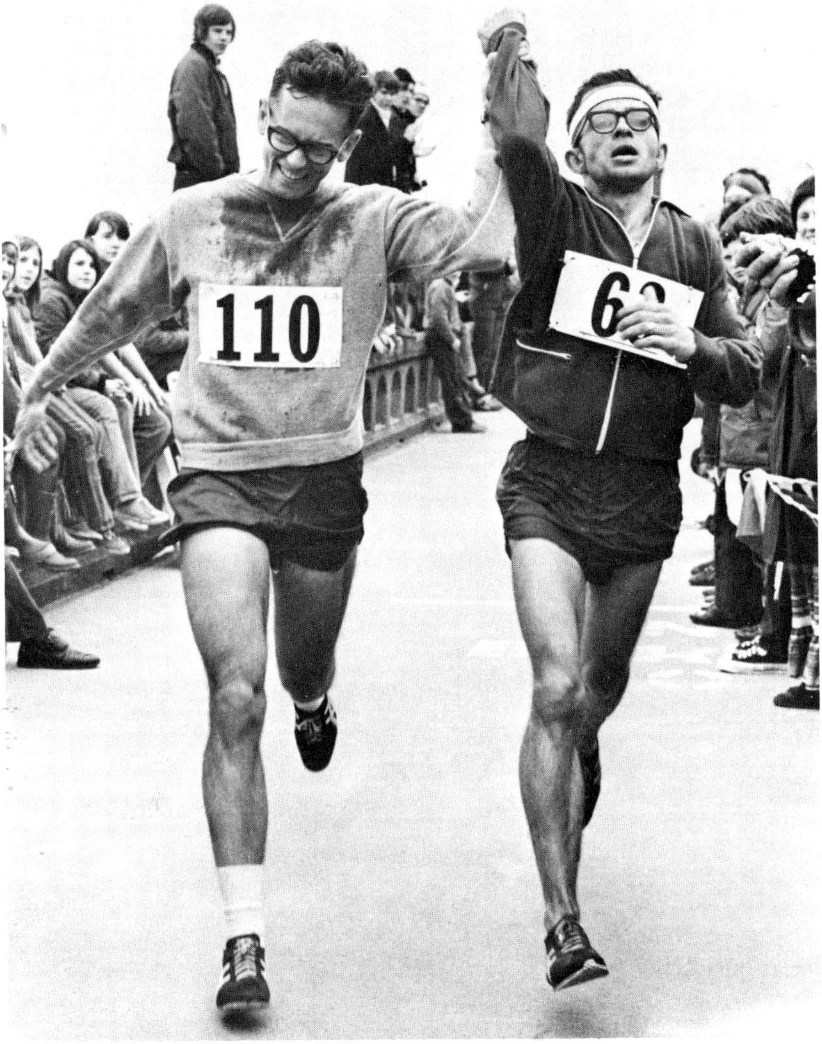

Shared pleasure at overcoming pain. (Bill Herriot photo)

COMMON INJURIES AFFECTING RUNNERS AND HURDLERS
STRAINS – SPRAINS – INFLAMMATION

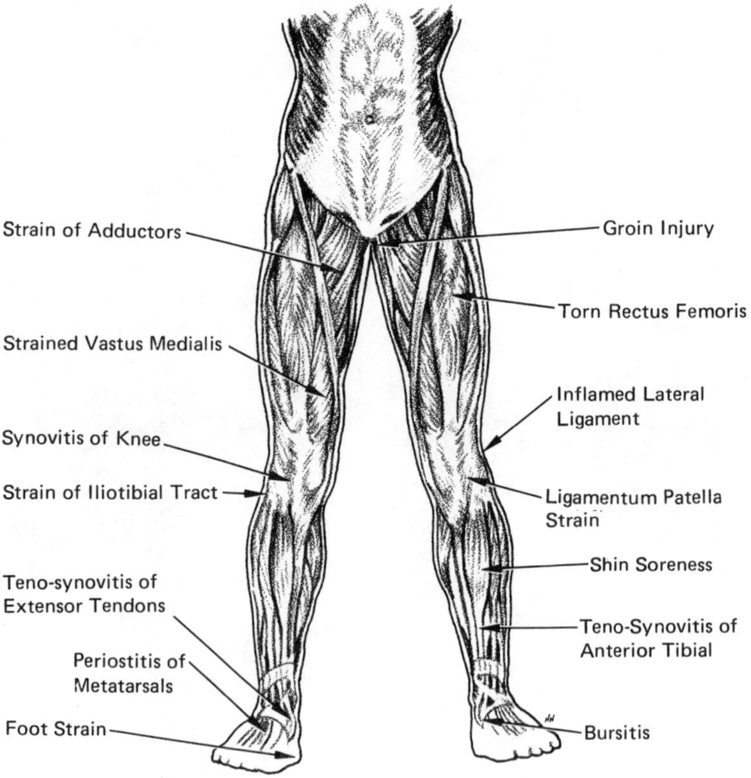

Reprinted from "Strength, Power and Muscular Endurance" by John Jesse

COMMON INJURIES AFFECTING RUNNERS AND HURDLERS

STRAINS – SPRAINS – INFLAMMATION

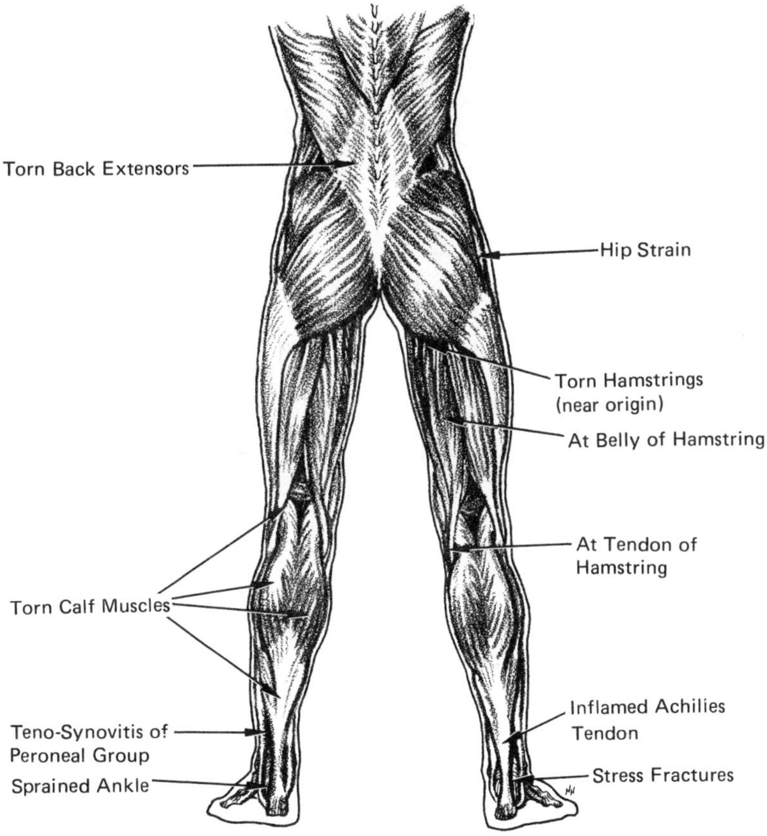

Reprinted from "Strength, Power and Muscular Endurance" by John Jesse

PAINS FROM THE BACK

Not only do many leg troubles start in the feet and work their way up. They also start in the lower back and migrate downward.

A case in point is sciatic nerve pain. This type of pain may originate in the lower back, even without overt symptoms in that area. The pain may be felt on down the course of the sciatic nerve, which travels along the back of the leg. Sciatic ailments are often incorrectly diagnosed as hamstring or calf "pulls" because of these symptoms.

Low-back and sciatic complaints are common. British researcher J.S. Lawrence found that they are experienced by over half the adult population. X-ray evidence shows that lumbar disc degeneration is found in similar proportions.

There are two main types of low-back problems: (1) lordosis (swayback), and (2) spondylolisthesis (slippage of the pelvis on the spine). Each of these ailments appears to irritate the roots of the sciatic nerves, causing pain to travel downward.

Another cause for difficulty is the fact that (according to one prominent researcher), 15% of the low-back-pain patients are found to have one leg shorter than the other. This throws the spine slightly out of alignment, and again may irritate the sciatic nerve root.

Long-range treatment must involve the detection and correction of basic problems. In the case of one leg being shorter than the other, inserting a heel lift under the short leg may give relief.

It appears that abdominal muscles are extremely important in the maintenance of a normal back. A good combination of abdominal muscles exercises is, for instances, situps and leg raises. *Avoid* hyperextension exercises (e.g., lying on the floor, belly down, and raising the head and legs simultaneously). These tend to make things worse.

The cure to root pressure is to reverse (or at least straighten) the curve of your back. Depending on the nature of the problem, heel lifts or abdominal exercises accomplish this. Some success has also been reported by athletes who have worn a belt-like "lumbo-sacral" support on their lower back.

Reference: *J. S. Lawrence, Annals of the Rheumatic Diseases, 28/121, 1969.*

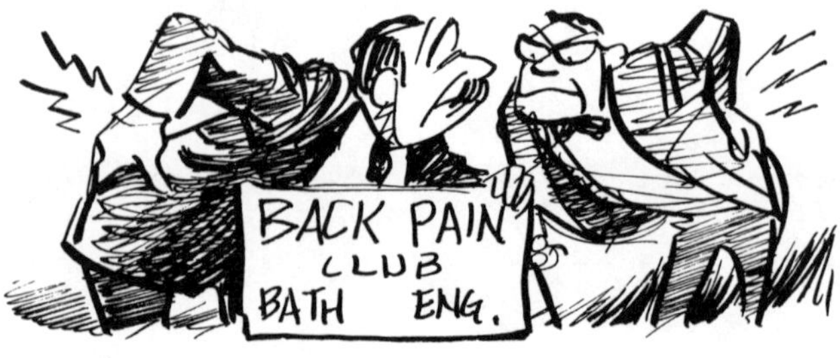

LEG MUSCLE PULLS

A theory on muscle pulls is gaining increasing support. It is that pulls—which in reality are tears or strains of the muscle fibers—result from an imbalance in muscular development.

Runners repeat the same action hundreds, even thousands, of times during a day's run. Since every stride is basically like every other, some muscles struggle while others coast. What happens is that the hard-working muscles get super-strong, while the "lazy" ones are neglected.

Sprinters appear to be particularly susceptible to such imbalances because of the explosive work they do. The quadriceps (front thigh) and hamstring (back thigh) muscles are the chief targets of injury. (Calf problems bother distance runners more often.)

Lee Burkett of San Diego State College tested a group of professional football players from the San Diego Chargers and trackmen from San Diego State. He measured them for relative strengths of their upper leg muscles. There were two sets of tests: one measured the strength of the muscles that extended the leg vs. those which flexed it; the other measured the difference in one leg vs. the other.

Burkett identified significant imbalances in six of the athletes and predicted they would pull hamstrings. Within three weeks of this prediction, four of the six did just that. Another one felt soreness in the predicted leg. He was assigned corrective exercises and had no further trouble.

Corrective exercises are designed to build up the weakened muscle to regain a balance.

Physiotherapist Joseph Zohar of New York, who works with college and professional athletes, advises corrective exercises both for the prevention and treatment of muscle pulls.

"The preventive exercise programs are meant primarily to supplement, not replace, conventional conditioning methods for healthy athletes," Zohar writes. "However, they should serve as a complete replacement following an injury. In treating an injured athlete, it is important to exercise not only muscles in the injured area, but also all other muscles which may affect it.

"I worked with a group of trackmen, all runners, from Adelphi University. One of them was Clyde McPherson, who ran in the US-Russia track meet in 1972. All but one of the runners had recurrent hamstring injuries. After only five sessions in my office, coupled with home exercises, their hamstring problems all but disappeared. I continued the program at my office for two or three more weeks, and then changed to a long-term maintenance program."

Zohar adds that "to help prevent injuries and strains, muscles must be strengthened and stretched to levels above the normal requirements of the sport. It is abnormal pulls and abnormal strains and stresses that produce injuries."

References: *A. J. Worthington, Modern Athlete and Coach, May-June 1971; Lee Burkett, Medicine and Science in Sports, Vol. 2 No. 1, Spring 1970.*

MUSCULAR CRAMPS

Muscle pulls apparently result from one kind of imbalance. Muscle cramps result from another. Cramping—which is usually, but not always, associated with hot weather running—comes on when a runner's fluid and electrolyte reserves have been severely drained.

Electrolytes are the minerals in the tissues. We think of common salt as being the key. But sodium chloride deficiency is only one of many factors. The runner also loses potassium, calcium and magnesium. Each of these substances is available naturally in food, and in commercial supplements.

When cramping occurs frequently it may be worthwhile to check for these dietary deficiencies. Getting adequate supplies of these minerals is important, along with getting enough water. And they have to be taken together. Replacing lost liquid only solves half the problem, as does replacing only lost electrolytes.

As a runner becomes conditioned to running itself and to running in hot weather, cramps should be less of a problem since the acclimatized runner's sweat contains a smaller percentage of salts.

References: *Runner's World, November 1971; David Costill, Distance Running News, September 1969.*

Dr. Kenneth Cooper has determined that magnesium deficiency is the major cause of muscle cramping in long distance runners.

Some of the magnesium is lost through sweating. But in a test of runners in Montana, Dr. J. Karr Taylor determined that the stools may be most responsible.

"Each runner ran at varying distances and saved stool for a week at each distance," Dr. Taylor reported. "In almost every case, there was a rather remarkable step-wise increase in the loss of magnesium via the stool—not the sweat."

He added, "It seems at least possible that the stool is the major avenue of magnesium loss in long distance runners, and the actual presence of intraluminal magnesium may well explain the observed absence of constipative difficulties in distance runners."

Taylor recommended that runners with cramping problems supplement their diets with a magnesium-protein complex called Magnesium Plus. He said many other magnesium preparations produce diarrhea, thereby compounding the problem.

Reference: *Runner's World, March 1972.*

Chapter Three

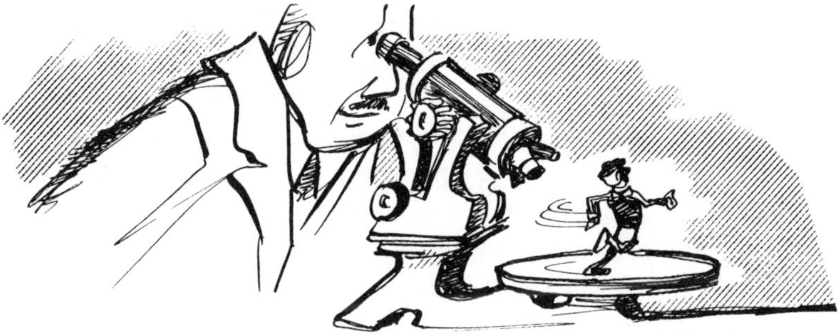

Internal Problems

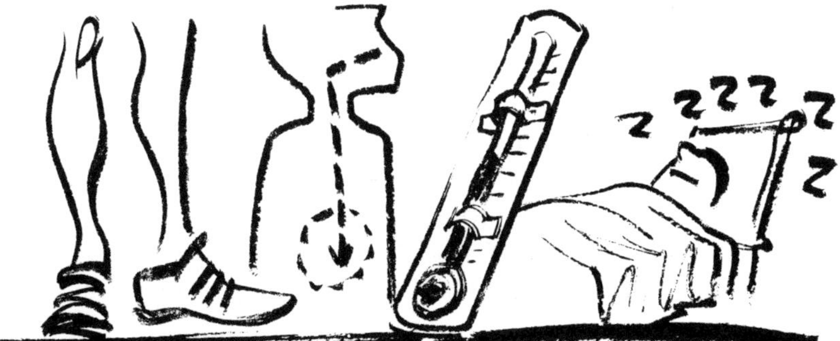

INTRODUCTION

Internal disorders work more subtly than external ones, but can be just as damaging. Since they're less obvious, the internal workings are more of a mystery. While it may be clear why a foot or a knee gets sore, it isn't so easy to pin down the causes and cures of a "stitch," post-race vomiting, or mononucleosis.

This chapter centers on the ailments of the cardiovascular, respiratory and digestive systems—which, to say the least, are complicated. Again, we add the disclaimer that (1) conclusions here are tentative, and (2) they center on the primary complaints of runners; one chapter can't be all-inclusive.

Mail received for the "Medical Advice" column in Runner's World indicates that the following are the most common "internal" complaints among runners:

- Severe stomach or intestinal pains while running—the most common of which is called "stitch."
- Weight control.
- Diarrhea and/or vomiting—usually associated with racing tension and exertion.
- After-effects from three illnesses: colds, flu and mononucleosis.
- Allergies such as hay-fever or asthma.
- Breathing difficulties (often associated with the allergies above).
- Heart-pulse "abnormalities."

Causes of this diverse collection of problems can't be summarized in a single sentence. But a majority appear to result from (1) overwork; (2) individual weaknesses; (3) dietary sources; (4) "normal" or "natural" occurrences.

Diet and nutrition are topics too big to tackle here. Another booklet in this series covers the "healthy" aspects of nutrition. For now, the discussion is limited to the dietary factors which plainly inhibit performance.

By realizing that some internal happenings are common—even healthy—runners may worry less about them.

MYSTERIOUS "MONO"

When Prince Albert died of typhoid, the disgruntled British press—according to Dr. Alex Comfort the expert on aging—referred to medicine as "the withered arm of science."

If that attitude is still prevalent among the general populace, one of the reasons is infectious mononucleosis—the "kissing disease." This disease continues to stump the experts while it hits the healthiest segment of our population, the young adults—and the healthiest segment of that group, the young athletes.

The boys in the white lab coats are getting desperate. They have been unable to satisfy the rules of their own infection game, rules known as Koch's postulates: (1) Find the bug; (2) Give the bug to a volunteer who gets the disease; (3) Retrieve the bug.

They have a prime suspect in the bug department called the EB virus. But they can't get past Step 2. Not even kissing will give it to a volunteer. My guess is that nothing will until they move their experiments out to the athletic field. They may have the right virus, but what they don't have is exhaustion.

Exhaustion is the key. Mono may be a virus disease. ("I am of the opinion," writes Dr. Betty Jo White in *Infectious Diseases,* "that the patient has the virus with him forever.") It may even be an auto-immune disease where the patient reacts to his own body (which was suggested by the late hematologist William Dameshek). But it rarely exists and almost never recurs without exhaustion.

Coaches are proving that every day. Wherever you find a team heading for regional or national ranking you are likely to find mononucleosis hitting the stragglers. Wherever you find champions on a squad, you are likely to find others in the infirmary.

Coaches must learn to individualize (and runners who coach themselves must learn to coach *themselves*—not some ideal runner their age) about hard work.

Hard work is not always bad. Some runners can accept it and become champions. Other would-be champions are destroyed by it. The coach who lumps his athletes together and gives uniform workouts will prove Darwin's "survival of the fittest" and wreck his team.

What happens may be called mononucleosis. Some call it staleness. Some call it "peaking too soon." But the symptoms are the same, and so are the effects: fatigue, swollen glands, poor attention span, restless sleep, bad performances. The bad performances are characteristic. The runner may suspect all is not right, but the initial part of the race holds no hint of disaster. Only in the last one-fourth of the race, as Yale coach Bob Giegengack observed, does the runner come apart. When he reaches back for the final lift, he finds he has nothing left.

Mono symptoms range from failure only under race conditions to an acute febrile illness with such problems as sore throat, tonsillitis, loss of appetite, jaundice, rash, and joint pains. Such an episode may also have occurred in the runner's past, with or without confirmation in a "mono-test."

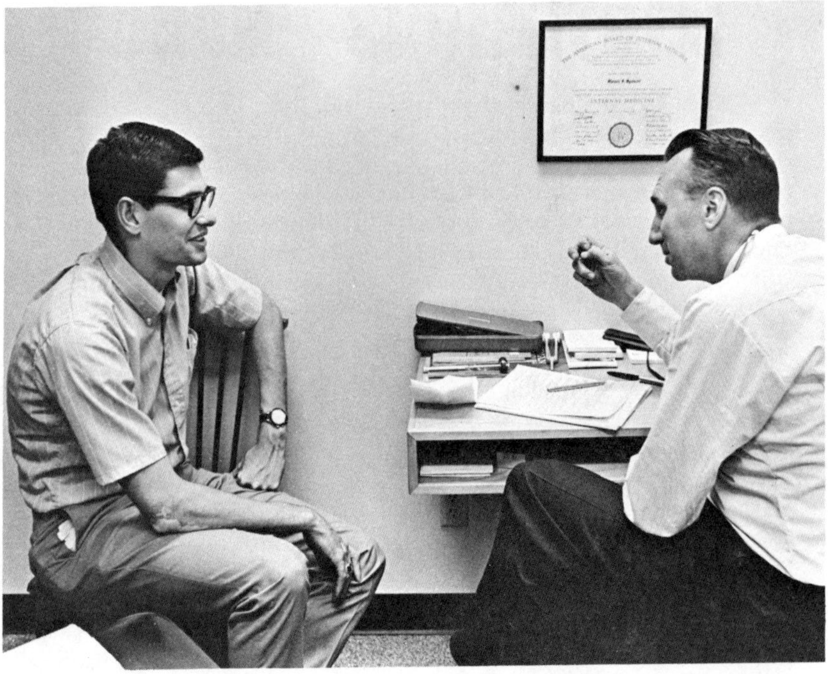

The runner's best friend may be his doctor. Jim Ryun, a man of many ailments, talks with his physician. (Rich Clarkson photo)

Some physicians claim one attack gives you a lifelong immunity against catching the disease again. If so, runners are not getting new attacks but relapses of their old disease. It is true that when symptoms return (usually in milder form) the "mono-test" is not positive. But runners certainly recognize their state as similar in kind, if not degree, with the mono attack.

Perhaps all we can say is that exhaustion in a certain group of individuals can cause a "mono-like" state. The treatment is rest, then every-other-day easy workouts until zest and the desire to train are regained—and workouts again become enjoyable. The temptation to race and find out whether one is well again should be resisted as long as possible.

Reduced activity and tincture of time are the essentials in the treatment of this disease.

COLDS AND THE FLU

Running can affect colds or "flu" one of two ways—direct opposites.

- When fitness and reserves are maintained at a high level, some protection against these ailments is noted. Runners may run right through the worst epidemics, being exposed constantly, without feeling a thing.

- But when the work load is particularly heavy and reserves lag, runners may be even more susceptible than the general population.

Colds and flu—along with mononucleosis—are stress related. It isn't the intent here to explore these illnesses deeply. But reviewing the Chapter One articles on stress will indicate how to avoid them.

Once they strike, though, the question becomes how to recover. This has to be an individual matter, since neither the patient nor the diseases are standardized.

As long as no fever is present, it appears safe to "run through" colds—taking care to run within the limits of energy and comfort and to stay warm. Gentle exercise tends to break up the congestion quicker than complete rest does. But keep the pace down so as not to induce coughing.

Colds with fever, and cases of the flu, require more delicate care. A period of convalescence—first rest, then a gradual return to a full schedule—is a must. Don't run with a fever. After that, as a rule of thumb, take two days easy for each day of fever. A week of fever and symptoms would need an additional two weeks' recovery period. Exhausting practices should be avoided at this time or recurrence is a distinct possibility.

Reference: *George Sheehan, Runner's World, March 1972.*

DIETARY DISORDERS

The aim of the ideal diet is to provide adequate calories with a proper proportion of protein (11-12%) and fat (35%) and recommended daily requirements of vitamins. Such a diet, according to J. V. Durnim, gives the athlete a "purely neutral environment." Along with most physiologists, Durnim does not believe fitness can be increased by diet. However, the wrong diet can cause trouble.

What we must learn are our own individual idiosyncrasies and food intolerances. We may not be able, for instance, to handle some of the following:

- **Milk**: 9% of Caucasians and a high percentage of Greek Cypriots, American Negroes, Arabs and Ashkenazi Jews cannot digest milk sugar. Another one percent have milk allegry. Most of these individuals have always avoided milk and should be encouraged to follow that body wisdom.

- **Gluten**: A protein found in all grains except corn and rice; found, therefore, in most cereals and baked goods; causes cramps, bloating, belching, diarrhea.

- **Highly Allergic Foods**: Chocolate, shellfish, strawberries, pork, melon, nuts, citrus fruits, egg white; cause stomach pains, diarrhea, bloating, rash, itching, headaches, nasal stuffiness, migraine headaches, etc.

- **Excessive Roughage**: Runners with spastic colons have trouble with raw fruit, raw vegetables, nuts, corn, beer, baked beans, cabbage, etc.; cause gas, bloating, pain, thin cigar-like or pencil-like stools.

- **Coffee**: Causes hyperacidity and stomach spasms in some people; also creates spasm in people with sensitive or irritable colons.

INTERNAL TURMOIL

Disorders in the digestive tract present a large variety of symptoms, and come from an even larger variety of causes. Because of their nature, they seem to strike at the most inopportune moments–namely before, during, and/or after races.

The digestive tract disturbances fall into three main categories as far as the runner is concerned:

- **Diarrhea.**
- **Vomiting.**
- **Stomach or intestinal pain.**

In all three cases, the emotional and physical stress of racing seems to bring them out. This indicates, apparently, that the cause is as much in the nerve centers of the brain as in the gut.

Diarrhea is a common pre-race symptom—so common, in fact, that it could almost be called "normal." It accompanies nervousness, as do increased urination and sweating.

Diarrhea becomes a serious consideration only when it is prolonged enough to cause dehydration or electrolyte deficiency (see accompanying article on dehydration, and muscle cramping section in Chapter Two.) Also, of course, there can be obvious problems if it occurs in mid-race.

When diarrhea strikes without the normal stress of racing, intestinal illnesses or food intolerances should be suspected.

Vomiting follows a similar pattern. It usually occurs after a strenuous effort (though it may happen before, or even *during*). Vomiting is a product of some combination of the following factors:

1. **Food intolerances** (see list on page 60).

2. **Fluid-electrolyte imbalance** (see articles on dehydration and muscle cramps).

3. **Acidity** (high levels of lactic acid in the system).

4. **Nerves** (the emotions of hard effort).

Stomach and intestinal pains are more serious considerations because they're most likely to directly influence running. These can be due to some of the same factors as diarrhea and vomiting. (And others—such as "stitch"—may not be related directly to the digestive process.)

Persistent internal pains may be an indication of uclers. Since ulcers are said to afflict 5% of the population and occur most often in the thin, ascetic type of individuals which make up the bulk of the distance running set, we might expect to hear about a high number of runners with such problems.

However, the incidence is low—apparently less than average for the general population. So rather than causing ulcers, running actually may lessen chances of having them.

Considering the alternatives, runners with ulcers can usually continue running if they do so cautiously. They naturally should work out a program in cooperation with a physician and keep a close watch on blood count (an indication of whether or not the ulcer is bleeding), on diet and on their total stress load.

THE "STITCH" DILEMMA

"Stitch" is a vague term applied to any number of internal pains that occur while running. A true stitch is a stabbing pain near the bottom of the rib cage. When it hits–it hits most often in the middle and latter portions of a distance race–the runner can't usually shake it until he has cut his pace.

Certain individuals are "stitch prone." They get these pains repeatedly in their races, much to their chagrin. On the other hand, others never have this problem though they race and train under exactly the same conditions.

Stitch susceptibility is still something of a mystery, but medical men have fairly well pinned it down to being a spasm of the diaphragm.

The spasm may be due to (a) unusual sensitivity to oxygen debt; (b) faulty breathing; (c) inherent weakness in the diaphragm; or (d) unaccustomed stretching. We're still grasping at straws when attempting to solve the stitch dilemma. But solutions might take these possible factors into account.

- The first two are related. Most stitches occur well into runs demanding high oxygen consumption and prolonged heavy breathing. Conscious attempts to breath regularly and deeply may reduce the possibility of spasm.

- Breathing exercises may help correct weaknesses in the diaphragm. Practicing running under the same conditions experienced in races may also develop a tolerance.

- A key factor appears to be unaccustomed stretching applied to an inherently weak diaphragm. This stretching comes in the form of heavy breathing, which is obvious. But a less obvious factor is hills. A startlingly high percentage of stitches strike while runners are going downhill. In theory, this is because they lean back while going down, and this puts strain on the diaphragm. If this is the case, attempting to lean forward might help.

Arthur Lydiard, among others, has suggested that stretching exercises aimed at the midsection are helpful for chronic stitch sufferers.

SUSPICIOUS URINE

The sight of blood in the urine understandably is a cause for concern among runners.

Blood in the urine is, however, a common result of exhausting work—particularly with long distance runners. One study revealed microscopic evidence of blood in the urine of 50-80% of long distance runners tested.

Traces of urine following hard endurance work very rarely has any clinical significance. It is seldom a sign of internal damage. Should it occur, though, with regularity and even in the absence of exhausting runs, medical advice should be sought.

In this same connection, runners also notice that their urine is a deep yellow color following strenuous runs. This is an equally innocuous symptom. The body is simply throwing off waste products accumulated during exercise.

References: *George Sheehan, Runner's World, November 1970; Philip Freedman, Sports and Physical Fitness/JAMA Questions and Answers.*

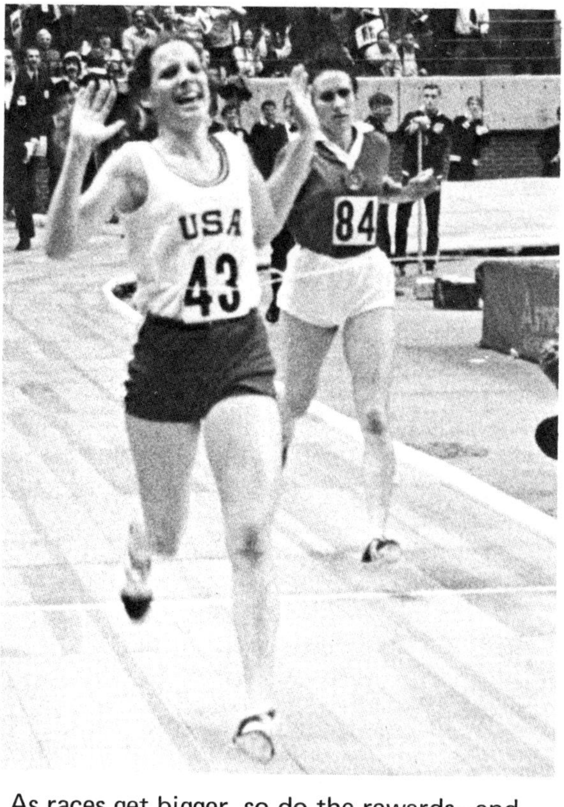

As races get bigger, so do the rewards—and the injury risks. (Penny Crowell photo)

CHRONIC DEHYDRATION

Liquids are lost much faster than they're replaced. In hot weather, this discrepancy is exaggerated, resulting in temporary or even chronic dehydration.

The effects of dehydration have been described by running researcher David Costill. "Generally speaking," Costill says, "when a man loses 2% or more of his body weight by sweating, his ability to perform prolonged exhaustive exercises is drastically impaired."

The crux of the problem, Costill notes, is that "regardless of how much a runner drinks, it will be impossible for him to keep up with the weight being lost by sweating."

Costill tested marathoners in the 1968 Olympic Trials. He found that the average weight loss was 9.3 pounds. Runners replaced only one-half pound of this loss during the race. In Costill's words, they only temporarily satisfied their thirst. He says that such partial replacement of liquids in long distance runners can, when they're training and racing hard in hot weather, lead to chronic dehydration.

"Large body water losses incurred on consecutive days may cause an accumulated weight and fluid loss. Man generally relies on his thirst to control body fluid balance. Unfortunately, this mechanism is far from accurate. In laboratory tests that required about eight pounds of sweat loss, we found that thirst was temporarily satisfied by drinking as little as one pound of water. Total replacement of body weight may take several days unless the runner forces himself to take more than desired."

Costill adds that chronic dehydration can drastically damage a runner's endurance capacity by lowering his tolerance to fatigue, reducing his ability to sweat, elevating his rectal temperature and increasing the stress on his circulatory system.

"Probably the best way to guard against chronic dehydration," he says, "is to check your weight each morning. If you should notice a two- or three-pound decrease from morning to morning, efforts should be made to increase your fluid intake. You need not worry about drinking too much fluid, because your kidneys will unload the excess water in a matter of a few hours."

Reference: *David Costill, Distance Running News, September 1969.*

RUNNERS' WEIGHTS

Two factors that simply don't go together are fast running and fat bodies. A recent survey of several hundred leading male runners—leading contenders for the 1972 US Olympic team—produced the following results:

- *Sprinters (100-440 yards) and hurdlers* showed average weights about normal for their height and age-group.

- *Middle-distance runners (880 yard to six miles)* averaged 11 pounds below American norms.

- *Long-distance runners (above six miles)* were 23 pounds below national averages.

- *Race walkers (20 and 50 kilometers)* were somewhat heavier than marathon runners but were still 14 pounds under normal levels.

Several conclusions can be drawn from these figures. Mainly, (1) the non-athletic American public is generally overweight, but (2) even when compared with "ideal" weight figures runners are on the light side, and (3) the longer the distance being run, the higher the energy demands and the less muscle bulk needed; hence, runners at longer distances burn off more weight and carry less bulk.

Although women weren't included in the study, the same conclusions probably would apply to them.

The accompanying charts compiled by the Metropolitan Life Insurance Company, list "average" weights for various ages and "desirable" weights for men and women ages 25 and over. (In theory, we cease growing in the early 20s, and should maintain a constant weight from that age on up.) Persons with small or medium frames are the ones most likely to be attracted to running in the first place.

A study of 500 leading distance runners (880 and up) indicates that typical running weight (in pounds) is approximately twice a man's height (in inches). In other words, at 5'8" (68-inch) man wouldn't vary much from the 136-pound figure. (Women average about 5% lighter for their height.)

Ernst Van Aaken, a German physician and coach, recommends that distance runners reduce themselves to 20% below average for the individual's height, frame and age. He says one of the primary values—if not the main benefit—of regular and extensive running is to shed weight and keep it off.

Not everyone's basic physical construction allows for weights as low as the "height-times-two." Nor will everyone have the psychological makeup that allows them to reduce as severely as Van Aaken suggests. But it is clear that weight control is a vital issue in the success of every runner. Weight and performance are directly related. Keeping routine records of both is a worthwhile practice.

References: *Runner's World, November 1971; Track & Field News, 1 March 1972; Statistical Bulletin, Metropolitan Life Insurance Company, November-December 1959.*

CONTROLLING WEIGHT

Does running reduce weight? It does and yet it doesn't. Running can put the weight in line, but it has to be combined with sensible dietary control.

Running alone accounts for approximately a 100-calorie energy expenditure per mile. A 10-mile workout equals 1000-1200 calories. It's simple arithmetic. If the runner thinks, "Now that I'm running, I can eat 2000 extra calories," he's working against mathematical reason. And he's going to stay heavy.

On the other hand, if caloric intake remains constant or is reduced, weight will go down accordingly. There is one point at which everyone can and will lose weight. Unfortunately, for some individuals, this can be as low as 300-500 calories per day.

Recent experimental work shows that with total fasting, individuals quickly lose weight. However, during short-term fasting, the major portion of weight loss is not fat but protein and water. The net effect is to reduce strength and throw off the body's water balance rather than trimming fat.

Exercise combined with caloric control eliminates this pitfall. When weight reduction is accomplished with exercise, there is a "muscle-sparing" action, with most of the weight loss being fat. (It has been estimated that one-half the loss would be muscle if you were only dieting.)

Since it takes about a 3500 calorie loss to lose a single pound, the burn-up through running may not appear significant. But multiply 500-1000 calories a day times 365 to get a better picture of potential year-long weight loss. Dieters must take such a balanced, gradual, long-term view.

Where there is an excess of fat, it will gradually diminish with the fattest parts clearing last. Most often this is around the waistline, hips and thighs. These deposits will be highly resistant to clearing until a person is down to absolutely lean weight.

References: *Journal of the American Medical Association, 211/3, 1970; Sports and Physical Fitness/JAMA Questions and Answers.*

AVERAGE WEIGHTS (MEN)

Height	15-16	17-19	20-24	25-29	30-39	40-49	50-59	60-69
5′0″	98	113	122	128	131	134	136	133
5′1″	102	116	125	131	134	137	139	136
5′2″	107	119	128	134	137	140	142	139
5′3″	112	123	132	138	141	144	145	142
5′4″	117	127	136	141	145	148	149	146
5′5″	122	131	139	144	149	152	153	150
5′6″	127	135	142	148	153	156	157	154
5′7″	132	139	145	151	157	161	162	159
5′8″	137	143	149	155	161	165	166	163
5′9″	142	147	153	159	165	169	170	168
5′10″	146	151	157	163	170	174	175	173
5′11″	150	155	161	167	174	178	180	178
6′0″	154	160	166	172	179	183	185	183
6′1″	159	164	170	177	183	187	189	188
6′2″	164	168	174	182	188	192	194	193
6′3″	169	172	178	186	193	197	199	198
6′4″	––	176	181	190	199	203	205	204

AVERAGE WEIGHTS (WOMEN)

Height	15-16	17-19	20-24	25-29	30-39	40-49	50-59	60-69
4′10″	97	99	102	107	115	122	125	127
4′11″	100	102	105	110	117	124	127	129
5′0″	103	105	108	113	120	127	130	131
5′1″	107	109	112	116	123	130	133	134
5′2″	111	113	115	119	126	133	136	137
5′3″	114	116	118	122	129	136	140	141
5′4″	117	120	121	125	132	140	144	145
5′5″	121	124	125	129	135	143	148	149
5′6″	125	127	129	133	139	147	152	153
5′7″	128	130	132	136	142	151	156	157
5′8″	132	134	136	140	146	155	160	161
5′9″	136	138	140	144	150	159	164	165
5′10″	––	142	144	148	154	164	169	––
5′11″	––	147	149	153	159	169	174	––
6′0″	––	152	154	158	164	174	180	––

IDEAL WEIGHTS (MEN)

Height	Small Frame	Medium Frame	Large Frame
5'2"	112-120	118-129	126-141
5'3"	115-123	121-133	129-144
5'4"	118-126	124-136	132-148
5'5"	121-129	127-139	135-152
5'6"	124-133	130-143	138-156
5'7"	128-137	134-147	142-161
5'8"	132-141	138-152	147-166
5'9"	136-145	142-156	151-170
5'10"	140-150	146-160	155-174
5'11"	144-154	150-165	159-179
6'0"	148-158	154-170	164-184
6'1"	152-162	158-175	168-189
6'2"	156-167	162-180	173-194
6'3"	160-171	167-185	178-199
6'4"	164-175	172-190	182-204

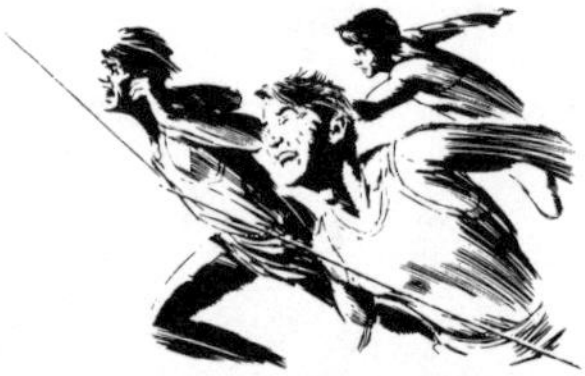

IDEAL WEIGHTS (WOMEN)

Height	Small Frame	Medium Frame	Large Frame
4'10"	92-98	96-107	104-119
4'11"	94-101	98-110	106-122
5'0"	96-104	101-113	109-125
5'1"	99-107	104-116	112-128
5'2"	102-110	107-119	115-131
5'3"	105-113	110-122	118-134
5'4"	108-116	113-126	121-138
5'5"	111-119	116-130	125-142
5'6"	114-123	120-135	129-146
5'7"	118-127	124-139	133-150
5'8"	122-131	128-143	137-154
5'9"	126-135	132-147	141-158
5'10"	130-140	136-151	145-163
5'11"	134-144	140-155	149-168
6'0"	138-148	144-159	153-173

HEART ATTACK DEATHS

To say that running provides absolute protection against heart disease is a gross oversimplification–if not entirely wrong. Claims for the heart-protecting qualities of running have had to be tempered somewhat as evidence of sudden attacks among apparently healthy joggers has come in.

John Cantwell, a physician at a federal penitentiary, treated three such cases–all prisoners who exercised regularly.

- **Case One**: A 38-year-old who jogged two miles nearly every day for two years. (He also smoked 2½ packs of cigarettes a day, drank 15 cups of coffee, and had a family history of heart disease.)

- **Case Two**: A 35-year-old who had jogged 2-5 miles a day for the past four months. (He also was a smoker, three packs a day, and was 20 pounds overweight. His father had died of a heart attack at age 42.)

- **Case Three**: A 35-year-old who had averaged an hour of handball a day for the past two years. (A two-pack-a-day smoker whose mother had died of a heart attack.)

Dr. Cantwell commented on these cases: "Vigorous physical exercise obviously did not protect the patients described herein from premature myocardial infarctions (heart attacks). Possibly the duration of exercise was not long enough. Perhaps exercise played a role in the patients' survival. In any event, exercise should not be overemphasized as a protective factor against coronary atherosclerosis. Indeed, it might even precipitate an acute event of the latter. Persons who exercise regularly should not be allowed to deceive themselves in reference to their overall health."

Another heart specialist, Meyer Friedman of San Francisco, has been quite outspoken in his opposition to strenuous running programs as heart conditioners–with good reason. Dr. Friedman has seen an increasing number of men die suddenly while they are running.

Friedman identifies a "Type A Behavior Pattern." Individuals with this type of personality, he says, are hard-driving, competitive, never-let-up types. "We're dead certain," he says, "that this type of personality is extraordinarily prone to coronary disease."

This is the way they approach their exercise, too–in a grim rush to get it out of the way. "This particular personality is a very peculiar one," Friedman notes. "It's extremely competitive and it is really hung up on the 'numbers racket.' Such individuals, if they do take up jogging, usually don't go for long distance running but allocate 15 to 30 minutes to do it. They have a miserable tendency to run the same distance daily, with the intent of increasing their speed."

These cases of sudden attack–even sudden death–among regular exercisers make several points:

1. That running itself isn't enough. Attention must be given to other factors in the life style.

2. That certain individuals have high inherited risk of heart disease. Running may have triggered the attack, but it just as easily could have occurred during any other strenuous activity.

3. That runners in it for the heart protection may be wise to slow down their pace and go longer. Short, violent bursts of running apparently create a greater risk and provide less conditioning than longer, gentler runs.

There are nine generally recognized risk factors that predispose an individual to heart disease: (1) high blood cholesterol; (2) high cholesterol diet; (3) high blood pressure; (4) cigarette smoking; (5) lack of activity; (6) overweight; (7) tension and stress; (8) diabetes; (9) family history.

Dr. Thomas Bassler, a Los Angeles medical examiner and distance runner, has reviewed the cases of hundreds of heart attack victims. He concludes that there are two categories of people in danger of attacks.

- *Acquired high risks*—"The usual picture of a coronary patient—overweight, smoker, sedentary and middle-aged."

- *Genetic high risks*—Those with inherited problems. "These genetic cases," Bassler says, "may not be overweight when they die. Often they are athletic and don't smoke."

He says about 8% of American men over 35 have "silent" coronary heart disease, and that sudden death is common during activities which build up oxygen debt or raise blood pressure sharply. Two out of three of these victims come from the "acquired risks," the other from the "genetic."

"There *are* a large number of 'jogging deaths,' " Bassler says, "if we include all men who die while wearing tennis shoes and performing any sort of exercise." He suggests that it is the *type* and *amount* of jogging or running that make the difference between precipitation and prevention of attack.

"Coronary heart disease," he notes, "is unknown in endurance type sports (like the marathon). I have never seen a case (myself or in the literature) of an arteriosclerotic coronary death in anyone who had finished a full marathon during the preceding six years. Marathoners have six years of protection, but anyone who is actively competing over the 10-kilometer distance also seems immune."

Dr. Bassler theorizes that a runner gets into this "protected" category only after he has logged about 1000 miles (i.e., enough training to handle a long distance race). He says the runner has to be able to do regular, yet slow, runs of six miles and more before he can begin feeling safe.

While testing his "Aerobics" program with the Air Force, Kenneth Cooper encountered an occasional death from heart attack. Over 15,000 men participated in one test. Two suffered heart attacks during the initial 12-minute run. (This part of the program was subsequently eliminated because of the tendency to race it while unfit.)

The testing continued with only minimal running—a mile or two a day. During the next six months, there were no further heart attacks.

Another 12,000 airmen from the same five bases weren't involved in the running program. During the same period, their group had nine heart attacks and two deaths.

Next Page: Men in their 40s, 50s and older are showing they can race successfully—if they recognize their limits. (George Beinhorn)

"So," Cooper says, "if you ask me how many people have been killed by aerobics and aerobic testing, I'll come right back and ask you how many people wouldn't be here today if they hadn't been exercising."

References: *J. D. Cantwell and G. F. Fletcher, Journal of the American Medical Association 210/130-131, 1969; Meyer Friedman, Runner's World, September 1971; Stampler and Blakeslee, Your Heart Has Nine Lives; Thomas Bassler, Runner's World, January 1972; Kenneth Cooper, Runner's World, September 1970.*

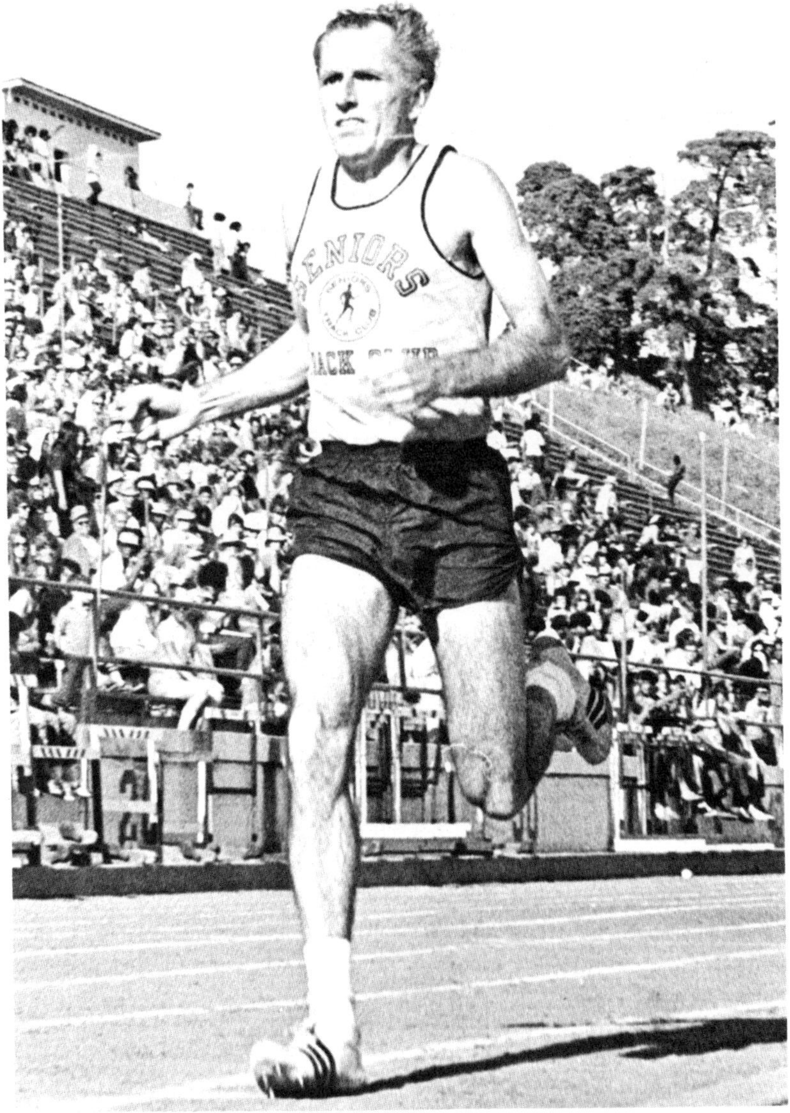

HEART "IRREGULARITIES"

The electrocardiogram machine's potential for interfering in an athlete's life was predicted from the work of Venerando and Rulli at the Rome Olympics.

The Italians studied a group of 89 world class marathoners and 38 walkers and found abnormalities (by current opinion) in almost all of them. Fully 12% had negative T-waves in the leads taken over the chest wall, a finding previously considered indicative of serious disease. Over 50% had abnormal conduction between the ventricles, and 15% had abnormally high electrical voltage. There were numerous other but less forbidding changes on the graphs.

The Venerando report suggested that any routine EKG screening of endurance athletes would turn up a number of odd and disturbing EKG tracings, and almost all these records could bother the usual electrocardiographer.

The prediction has come true, mostly because this report (along with another from Israel) has not reached general acceptance. It is difficult, you see, to conceive that changes usually connected with disease can occur in a heightened physiological state—which endurance fitness is.

Runners subjecting themselves to comprehensive physical examination (my advice is to get one for a baseline and then see a doctor only when you are sick) should be aware that their EKG may be misinterpreted.

It is well to remember Venerando's conclusion:

- The changes are not related to decreased heart function or disease.
- They are not accompanied by any heart enlargement beyond that physiological change associated with the sport.

Similar "normal abnormalities" have been reported with other groups of athletes.

- **Heart "Murmur"**—A test of one group of college lacrosse players indicated that 11 of 15 athletes had a "third sound" after exercising. Researcher Dave Lavine said the third sound is often thought to be indicative of heart disease, but "before being studied, the heart of each player was given a thorough cardiological physical examination. All had sound hearts. The murmurs developed *after* the hearts were well conditioned.

"At resting stage, a well-conditioned heart will pump more blood at a slower rate than normal, thus producing the murmur-type sound. Once an athlete is out of training, the murmur and sounds should disappear."

Lavine noted that doctors should recognize the "third sound" as a healthy one, and not to improperly diagnose it as a heart problem.

- **Palpitations or Irregular Pulse**—Irregular pulse or premature heart beats are rarely indicative of heart disease. They are usually due to constitutional diseases such as thyroid, allergy, or excessive use of stimulants. They are also sometimes seen as an exhaution symptom. Runners might do well to taper off training when they occur.

- **Slow Pulse**—Most runners are "vagotonic." Their vagus nerve which slows the pulse (as well as narrowing the pupils and increasing stomach acid secretions) is dominant. Slow pulse, down in the 50s, 40s, or even lower, is common and no cause for concern.

• **Low Blood Pressure**—Of itself it is no problem. But if blood pressure falls when a person stands, light-headedness or even fainting may occur. This state frequently is experienced when an athlete is training heavily. It is felt, like so many other unusual body signs, to be an exhaustion phenomenon and may mean the runner is at or passing his peak.

References: *Journal of Sports Medicine and Physical Fitness, September 1964; Dave Lavine, Perspective Correlation of Left Ventricular Performance with Murmurs and Sound in the Athlete's Heart.*

AMOUNTS OF SLEEP

Sleep not only regulates how much work a runner can do. It also is a sensitive indicator of overwork.

It is vital that the runner get a proper amount of sleep, but the definition of "proper" is a highly individual matter. Some individuals are "six-hour-people," while some are "10-hour-people." Either too little *or* too much is thought to reduce the energy level.

Recent research into the effects of sleep deprivation on work capacity is interesting. One test indicated that long periods of sleep deprivation do not alter performance. Short-term physical loads were handled better after 120 hours of sleep deprivation than with normal sleep. However, there was a gradual decline in mental performance. (The sleep-deprived subjects slept up to 20 hours straight after the test, then took up to three days to recover.)

Two other generally recognized facets of sleep should be mentioned:

• Sleep loss *two* nights before a hard run is more damaging than a shortage the night before.

• Some individuals operate best in the morning, while others wake up more slowly and don't hit their stride until later in the day.

The latter should be taken into account in the timing of daily runs. Research has shown that a "morning person" may be operating at full efficiency 15 minutes after he awakens, while a "night person" may not wake up fully for two hours.

Sleep disruption—difficulty in getting to sleep and staying asleep, particularly the latter—is a key sign of stress, and may indicate that you're overdoing in your running.

Reference: *George Sheehan, Runner's World, January 1972.*

EFFECTS OF DRUGS

BY MANFRED STEINBACH

This article by Dr. Steinbach, a German Olympic long jumper in 1964, is reprinted with permission of Australia's "Modern Athlete and Coach."

In 1962, a doping survey in Italy discovered appalling facts when 50% of amateur cyclists and 27% of footballers examined had been doped. It has been stated that 70 out of 100 cyclists in the "Tour de France" are using drugs in order to withstand the enormous strain. Likewise, this can be tempting for long distance runners, swimmers and rowers. Boxers, parachutists, high divers and racing drivers resort to drugs to muster up courage. Jumpers, throwers and weight lifters use hormones to improve explosive strength and reaction speed.

Many drugs, particularly those taken to improve endurance, can be dangerous to health and life. For example, a cyclist collapsed with poisoning symptoms during the world championships in 1961. Subsequent examination proved that a drug of the dangerous amphetamine variety had been taken. Dane Knut Jensen died during the 100-kilometer team race at the 1960 Olympic Games in Rome. Again it was proved that drugs had been taken. Recently, English cyclist Tom Simpson fell from his bicycle in a condition of absolute exhaustion in the 13th stage of the 1968 "Tour de France" and later died. "You can't win the Tour on water," three-time winner Louison Bobet commented.

Most sportsmen using drugs have wrong ideas as to the effects. An untrained sportsman can hardly replace lack of training by doping, nor can real crisis in performance capacity be balanced by drugs. Work physiology demonstrates that 20-30% of our maximum performance capacity remains inaccessible. This is known as the "autonomously protected reserve," which normally is released in moments of great emotion or excitement as an emergency function.

What actually bars access to this last reserve is the feeling of fatigue and the accompanying decrease in performance at the stage of work which is still well below physical exhaustion. Thus the fatigue occuring during a sporting activity is a warning signal. There is no relevant safety gap between fatigue and exhaustion. Under the effect of doping the boundaries can become so close that the doped athlete collapses in absolute exhaustion, often without warning symptoms.

By doping, subjective performance limits can be brought up to the level of objective performance limits. The doped endurance athlete feels no fatigue, has unimpeded access to the last physical reserves and thus endangers his life. Here the psycho-physical doping problem becomes apparent. The drugs eliminate the subjective and objective fatigue symptoms. They also create a condition of euphoria–elation not justified by reality–and prevent realistic orientation. This sometimes takes the character of intoxication or even semi-trance.

Inhibition, in addition to fatigue, also leads to doping practice. Athletes use drugs to overcome nervousness and excitement. Others, mostly insecure and neurotic, use it to eliminate inhibitions which can have an adverse effect on performance.

German sports doctors have suggested that doping is the use of any medicine to improve performances. According to the present definition, a cup of coffee is regarded as a generally accepted ingredient of nutrition but this does not apply to caffeine tablets or an overdosage of coffee. The problem is not only what substances are used but also the dosage. The use of oxygen, a physiological substance, apparently is not regarded as doping. But what about the method of supply, as for example inhalation from a cylinder, and the concentrated quantity?

Doping can be divided as follows:

1. Psychically effective substances, subdivided into stimulants and sedatives.

2. Substances affecting the circulatory and respiratory systems.

3. Substances affecting metabolism.

4. Substances affecting hormones.

The dangerous substances belong mainly to the first group, while other groups often contain preparations which can be classified as "doubtful."

• **Group 1**: Caffeine (from coffee and tea) and amphetamines excite the motor centers in the brain and radically remove fatigue symptoms. While amphetamines taken under medical supervision are administered in doses of a fraction of a gram, doping cases involving over 20 times the amount are known. Amphetamines play some part in almost all doping cases.

Tests with animals have shown that rats, whose lives are in danger, swim no better under the influence of amphetamines than they would otherwise in this situation. Other tests have indicated that while endurance is improved by amphetamines, coordination is impaired. Footballers, for example, play with better stamina, but their ball deliveries are inaccurate. In cycling, because the cyclist sits and is stabilized, pepping by amphetamines leads to the desired performance improvement. However, even at the least overdosage the danger of an overstrain is imminent.

Performance improvements can also be achieved with a slight consumption of alcohol and using narcotics, such as morphine, heroin, cocaine and hashish. Recently, psycho-drugs have been used to eliminate tension. Certain psycho-drugs are supposed to lessen stage-fright which can be detrimental to performance. But, as a certain amount of nervous tension is a prerequisite to top performance, the success of these relatively harmless drugs is doubtful.

• **Group 2**: This includes preparations which cause a widening of the blood vessels and possibly a better supply of blood to the muscles. Experimental examinations, however, have led to the conclusion that little or no improvement can be expected in healthy people.

The intake of pure oxygen economizes the work of the organism and provides favorable results in prolonged practices. The pulse rate, for example, is markedly lower during inhalation of oxygen. So far, technical difficulties have prevented constant use of oxygen and since oxygen can't be stored by the body there is no doping problem, except the psychological advantage of using it before competition.

• **Group 3**: Substances affecting metabolism are various sugars, vitamins, phosphates, proteins and mineral preparations. They certainly can improve performance of undernourished people, but are unnecessary to sportsmen under normal circumstances. An immediate improvement, after taking any of these substances, is extremely doubtful—except in cases of long periods of strain which leads to exhaustion of the existing energy stores, like in marathon or long distance cycle races.

Here it must be remembered that no significant digestion occurs during sporting activity, making the intake of such substances during the competition rather questionable. As long as foods are taken in the normal manner, it can not be regarded as doping. However, glucose injection must be rejected because it means supplying the body in an abnormal way.

• **Group 4**: This group includes a variety of hormones used to improve sporting performances. Among these is adrenalin, produced by the body in great physical and emotional tension to release energy reserves. Adrenalin would be a suitable means of doping, but its utilization in sport has so far failed. Finding the correct dosage is complicated, and excessive reactions occur easily and often. The hormones of the thyroid gland and female sex hormones have also proved unsuccessful,with the exception of the borderline case of postponement of menstruation by using hormones.

Proceeding from the fact that male sex hormones promote muscle growth and strength, these hormones have been adminstered with great success. Synthetic male hormones—anabolic steroids—activate protein metabolism, and experiments with Dianabol and similar products have shown a definite improvement in the muscle power. It is even possible to develop isolated muscles by direct administration of anabolic steroids to certain areas. The advantage of using male hormones (there have been enormous improvements in performances) leaves no doubt that the use of anabolic steroids should be classified as doping.

From the many preparations available, only a few have the desired affect. There is a small group of effective drugs, but most of these are dangerous to health. They mobilize the last reserves of the organism and block protective reactions of the body. If additional unexpected stresses occur, as in the case of high atmospheric temperatures of great humidity, the doped athlete is unable to summon his protective mechanism and the final results can be disastrous.

Chapter Four

Environmental Problems

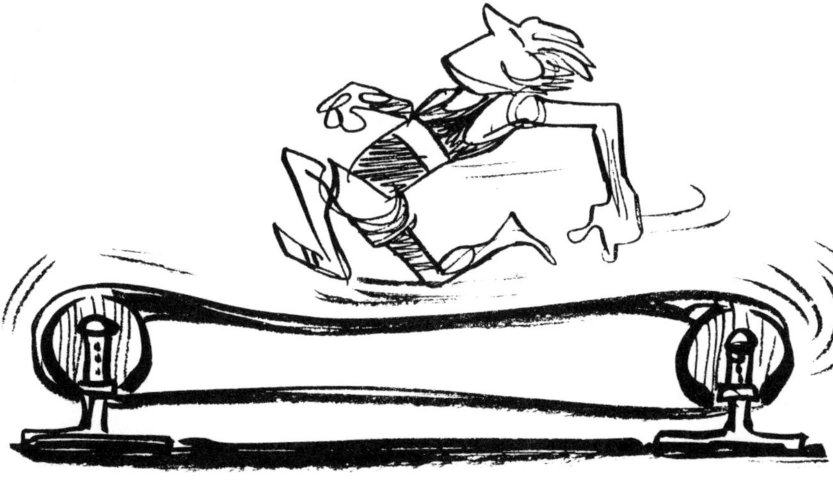

INTRODUCTION

It might be said that environmental factors are beyond our control. That's true. But we can control the way we REACT and ADAPT to these factors. Those reactions and adaptations are the key points of this chapter, which discusses the potential harmful effects of the external environment.

These environmental factors fall into five general categories:

- **Heat**—This is one of the few elements in running that can truly be a life-or-death matter. The long distance runner must learn to cope with hot weather and to recognize what it can do to him.

- **Cold**—It's less of a problem than heat. But exposure to severe cold can disrupt running, if not actually damaging health. If anything, however, runners probably treat cold too seriously and heat too lightly.

- **Storms**—The lightning and high winds of a thunderstorm can cause obvious problems to runners caught out in the open.

- **Air Pollution**—As cities become increasingly crowded, the problem of finding clean air (the fuel of running) becomes more critical.

- **Altitude**—The problem here is similar to that of air pollution—finding enough oxygen. But altitude alone isn't a health hazard. There is simply less oxygen available. This fact influences performances and requires that low-land athletes go through an adaptation period.

Heat, cold, air pollution and high altitude get some attention in this chapter, as they relate to the health and safety of the runner. Heat and cold are stressed because they are facts of every runner's life.

The runner may not be able to turn the environment off and on as he would an air conditioner. But if he's fit, and armed with awareness of environmental forces, they pose less of a threat.

HOT-WEATHER RUNNING

1. The best way to handle heat is (a) training in a hot atmosphere (Buddy Edelen trained in double sweats in damp, chilly England then won the 1964 Olympic marathon trial in 90-degree heat) and (b) being in good shape (veteran runner Aldo Scandurra has observed that many marathoners do well in cool weather with workouts averaging five miles a day, but hot weather races put them away).

2. Ten days to two weeks of hot weather training should stimulate the body to adapt by:

- Improving circulation to skin.
- Improving sensitivity and capacity of sweating mechanism (begin sweating at lower temperature).
- Reducing salt loss by kidneys and sweat.

3. Pre-race drinks (sodium chloride-potassium-sugar mixture) may be helpful. But the body quickly throws off excess so don't rely on this completely.

4. During races, assure adequate intake of cold fluids—preferably balanced sodium-potassium-sugar mixture (other minerals, especially magnesium, may also be shown to be necessary). South African researcher C. H. Wyndham recommends about 10 ounces every 30-40 minutes; amount can be determined from weight loss the runner usually has under such conditions.

Gatorade has very little potassium. Orange juice or slices are good sources of this mineral. *Sportade* seems to be the best commercially available drink, though *ERG* ("Gookinaid")—a new preparation—may be even better. Orange juice with a weak salt solution can be a good homemade solution.

5. Wearing a cap or knotted handkerchief helps with solar radiation. Dousing the head and trunk liberally at each water stop, and placing ice in the cap or down the back of the running shirt are also helpful. Care should be taken, however, not to get shoes wet, or blisters may result.

Heat can kill. It has killed in the past and will kill again, often without regard for a runner's ability. The best ones are as susceptible as the also-rans—and often more so since the former tend to drive themselves harder.

All runners and officials connected with distance racing should be acquainted with the symptoms and treatment of heat-related ailments.

There are two types or degrees—heat exhaustion, and heat stroke.

- **Heat exhaustion**—Collapse resulting from inadequate replacement of fluids or electrolytes. The symptoms are pale, clammy skin and normal to sub-normal temperature. Treatment involves fluid-electrolyte replacement.

- **Heat stroke**—This is far more serious and can cause death. In stroke, the skin is red and quite hot. Reduce the temperature *immediately*.

Be alert for a transition from exhaustion to stroke. If the exhaustion victim doesn't respond to treatment, rush him to a doctor.

Gabe Mirkin, a physician and marathoner, offers this advice on heat stroke. The warning symptoms include: (1) legs start to burn; (2) breathing becomes difficult and there's a buring in the chest; (3) head aches; (4) you feel dizzy; (5) when you slow down, it hurts even worse. "The warning of heat stroke," he says, "is that it does not feel better stopped, but feels worse."

Once a person has gone into heat stroke, Mirkin advises the following:

"Forget about giving the victim fluid by mouth. It is worthless. You are interested in cooling him immediately. His temperature may be 110. Evaporation is the key. Pour anything you can on the victim, immediately (water, milk, Coke, Gatorade, etc.). Rub his skin vigorously to open up the surface blood vessels. Hose water on him. The best thing to do is to rub ice cubes all over his body. Above all, keep pouring something wet on him."

References: *Fred Hurd, Runner's World, May 1970; Gabe Mirkin, Marathon Handbook 1972.*

"WET-BULB" TEMPERATURES

The present frenzy of devising bigger and better hardware to measure physical performance has failed to surpass a simple $12 instrument found in any physics laboratory—the wet bulb thermometer. It has been part of physics labs for decades. But no one thought to use it in athletics—until football players started to die of heat stroke.

Almost unknown prior to 1959, deaths then began to appear at the rate of 5-6 a year. These fatalities quite evidently related to heat and humidity, but the question was which was more important and what combination was dangerous. The wet bulb reading was found to give a single corrected humidity reading which could be correlated to clinical symptoms.

Physicians working with football teams found a reading of 80 to be dangerous and recommended frequent rests, light clothing and increased fluid and salt intake. The athlete's weight was also watched closely. Wet bulb values up and down the scale were discovered to require different levels of precautions.

It then became obvious that the value of the wet bulb reading for the distance runners was not only for survival but also performance. In marathons, heat and humidity provide a tremendous additional load—an additional variable that the runner must consider. It gives an advantage to those with more "bottom" or mileage background. Just like hills, wind or any additional ballast, it separates runners during a race. Premium is placed on judgment and pace because at no other time does an initial fast pace penalize a runner more.

A good example of this occurred in 1967 at Holyoke, Mass., in the trial for the Pan-American Games marathon. The race, subsequently known as the Holyoke Massacre, was won by Ron Daws, a steady marathoner, who ran 20th most of the way, and won almost by default when over 60% of the field dropped out (some of them literally).

It was the worst carnage since the "Inferno," the 1909 Boston Marathon run in 97-degree heat, in which 91 of 164 starters failed to finish and only the winner, Henri Renaud (who like Daws was well back at the halfway mark) finished the course without walking.

Finishing behind Daws at Holyoke were two outsiders, 43-year-old Jim McDonagh and Tom Osler, known to his racing colleagues as "the Turtle," declared that he had beat the heat.

One who didn't was the favorite, Tom Laris, runner-up at Boston and the reigning American marathoner. Laris had collapsed once before and, noting the onset of similar symptoms, he withdrew.

World class distance men can learn a lesson from some of their older colleagues. For years it has been known that older runners perform better comparatively than younger ones in hot, humid weather. It apparently is because they run without regard to the clock or who is near them, but just at what appears to be the correct pace.

The hotter and more humid it gets, the more crucial pacing becomes. The wet-bulb reading is a valuable guide to how far you can push.

The military now makes extensive use of Wet Bulb Globe Temperatures (WBGT)–limiting or even curtailing training when these readings climb above "safe" levels.

These temperatures are obtained from three different thermometers:

- A standard theremometer shaded from the sun.
- A black-globe thermometer exposed to the sun and prevailing wind.
- A stationary wet-bulb thermometer similarly exposed.

The WBGT, or "heat-stress index," is determined by adding seven-tenths of the wet-bulb reading, two-tenths of the black-globe reading, and one-tenth of the standard thermometer reading.

The military uses these figures as its guidelines.

1. WBGTs below 80 are relatively safe for vigorous physical activity.

2. When the WBGT hits 85 degrees, "only those people who have been exercising in the heat for at least *10* days can continue their workouts."

3. When the WBGT hits 88 degrees, "only those people who have been exercising in the heat for at least *30* days can continue vigorous outdoor workouts."

4. When the WBGT hits 90 degrees, "it is best for all individuals to *stop* vigorous outdoor exercise regardless of the state of conditioning or heat acclimatization."

Reference: *Kenneth Cooper, New Aerobics.*

On cold days like this one, the thinly-dressed runners stay more comfortable than the bundled spectators. (Steve Sutton photo)

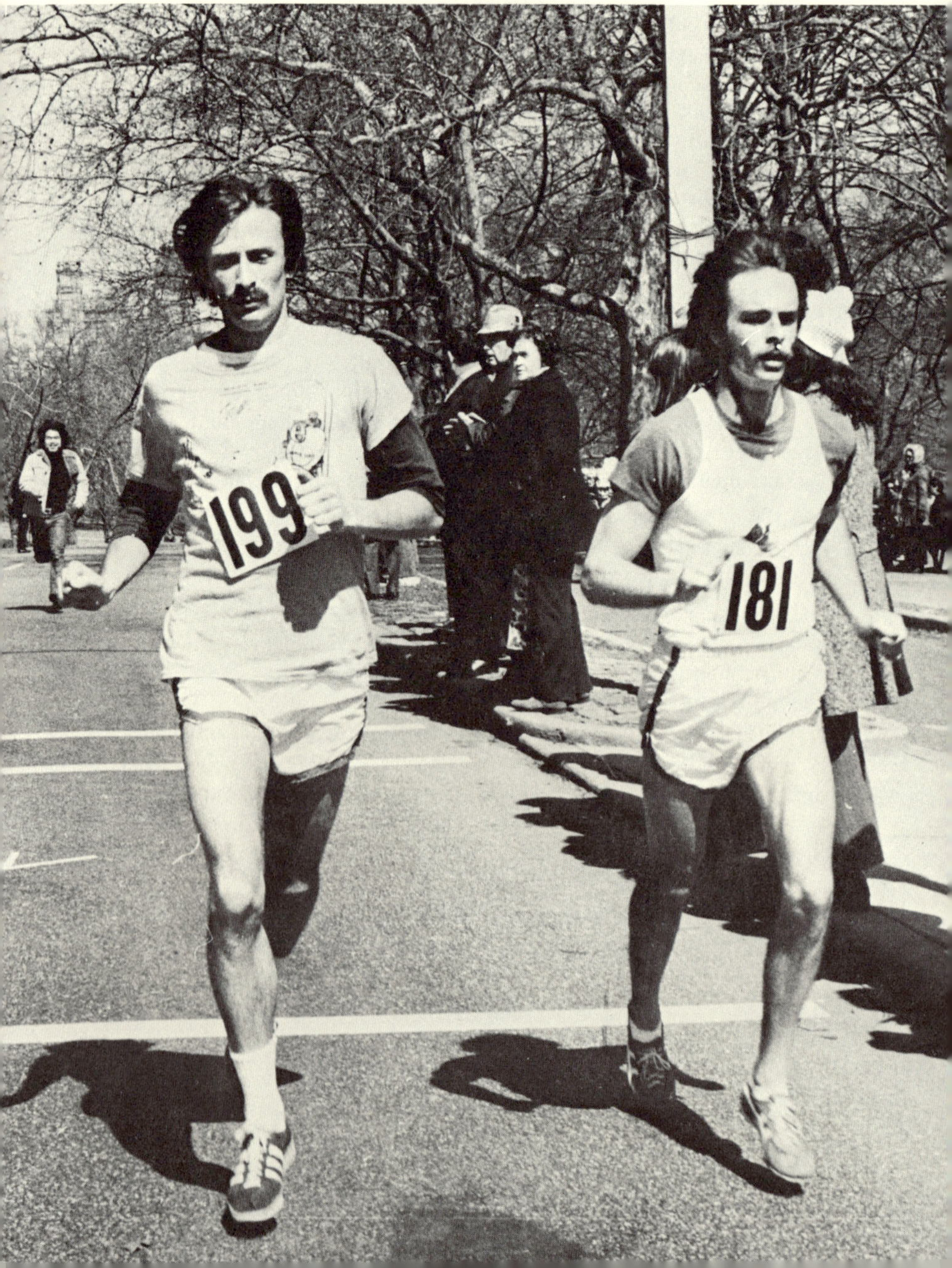

COMPENSATING FOR COLD

Cut Bank is a northern Montana community which regularly vies with such famous ice burgs as International Falls, Minn., and West Yellowstone for coldest spot in the nation. Several winters found me huddled in the fire; all advice and commonsense indicated this was only sanity. Twenty to 30 below zero is routine here, and even colder days are not unusual. As striking perhaps as the cold are the winds; 40-60 m.p.h. velocities are frequently experienced.

The training gap generated by this winter hiatus appeared unavoidable, but one winter my desire to run finally overcame my good sense. I ran through, and learned some things about extreme cold weather running that may help others.

WHEN TO RUN

There are inviolable limits to sensible and useful winter runnings. The wind-chill index probably is the best guide. The chart here shows the relative danger at various wind-chill levels.

I do not run if the wind-chill is in the red ("great danger"). In the yellow ("increasing danger"), I dress with special care. In the green ("little danger"), I run without fear.

Wind *direction* is critical. A side wind has but a fraction of the impact of a headwind. The trailing wind is important only if you have to return into it. Worth noting, too, is that to run into the wind at, say, 5 m.p.h. increases wind chill appreciably. A glance at the chart will show that this increment can easily push you out of the yellow into real danger.

Short distances also will minimize the effects of wind-chill. On very bad days, I split the workout (never over 12 miles).

WHAT TO WEAR

Here, too, one can use the wind-chill chart.

In the green, briefs, top and bottom thermal underwear, wool sox, nylon warmup pants, a hooded sweatshirt and mittens (or even less) suffice.

In the milder yellow, add a thermal shirt and knit pullover mask. The mask should have separate eyeholes (the bridge of the nose is prone to frostbite) and no mouth hole. If air exchange is impaired, fashion multiple vertical breathing slits. My frontal sinus area seems particularly sensitive to extremes of cold, so I pull the wool mask well down over the eyebrows.

In the nastier yellow, add thermal bottoms (this pair need not be full length), a second pair of mittens or gloves, and a leather mask. This mask can be carried handily and used only on the into-the-wind segments if desired. Sometimes plastic goggles can be used in place of the leather mask. They allow use of glasses without quite so much fogging (I have found no product completely satisfactory in keeping glasses clear).

Total maximum weight of clothing with shoes is about seven pounds, and with newly available lightweight nylon clothing could be even less.

Since wind-chill is a two-part index (cold and wind), its variables are frequently best combatted by adapting dress to the dominant factor. At -40 degrees and 5 m.p.h. (wind-chill=47) insulated cold-proof clothing is in order. At -10 degrees and 15 m.p.h. (wind-chill=45), wind-proof clothing should be considered.

HOW TO RUN

Without stopping and when possible exclusively with the wind.

WHERE TO RUN

On a well-traveled road or with a "flight-plan" known to someone who cares.

WHAT YOU'RE AVOIDING

• **"Cold Stress"**—A poorly defined climatologic insult, this stress contributes to the general (de)adaptation syndrome (GAS). In practice, it retards at least and exhausts at worst. Vitamin C (1000 mg. daily) has been recommended, but I have no personal use experience.

• **"Frostbite"**—Not always a minor insult, frostbite can maim, disable or kill. Adequate clothing and commonsense have minimized these risks of winter training, but with all precautions minor 'bite has so far seemed unavoidable. Further experience will probably provide complete protection.

• **"Lungburn"** is apparently a manufactured peril. At no time has my respiration been in any way painful or compromised. There does seem to be increased production of pulmonary mucus, but this is handled without difficulty.

WHAT YOU'RE ACCOMPLISHING

The triumph of beating wind-chills as low as -72 degrees is exhilarating. The benefits of continuous *and* comfortable training without that spring retraining strain are clear and satisfying.

TREATMENT OF FROSTBITE

Frostbite, which can occur at any temperature under 32 degrees, most commonly strikes the feet, hands, ears and nose—in that order. Protective measures are described in the accompanying article by Dr. Taylor.

If you think you have frostbite, take the following steps:

• **Rewarm rapidly**, but do not use excessive heat. Placing frostbitten feet in a warm oven or near an open fire may feel good temporarily, but it may also result in cold injury compounded by burn injury. The correct rewarming procedure is to use water at about body temperature (no higher than 104 degrees).

• **Do not walk on or massage the frozen part.** This could cause mechanical injury.

• **Do not rub with snow.** Both the cold of the snow and the mechanical rubbing intensify the injury.

• **Seek immediate medical treatment.**

There are four degrees of injury. First degree means no tissue loss; second degree is partial thickness skin loss; third degree is full thickness skin loss; fourth degree is loss of a part–skin, muscle and bone.

The assessment of degree, however, can only be made by a doctor. At first, all frostbite injuries appear the same: cold, pale and firm-to-hard to the touch. Treat all suspected frostbite as if it were a serious injury.

Reference: *Patient Care, November 15, 1971.*

Wind chill factor chart

Estimated wind speed (in mph)	Actual Thermometer Reading (° F.)											
	50	40	30	20	10	0	-10	-20	-30	-40	-50	-60
	EQUIVALENT TEMPERATURE (° F.)											
calm	50	40	30	20	10	0	-10	-20	-30	-40	-50	-60
5	48	37	27	16	6	-5	-15	-26	-36	-47	-57	-68
10	40	28	16	4	-9	-24	-33	-46	-58	-70	-83	-95
15	36	22	9	-5	-18	-32	-45	-58	-72	-85	-99	-112
20	32	18	4	-10	-25	-39	-53	-67	-82	-96	-110	-124
25	30	16	0	-15	-29	-44	-59	-74	-88	-104	-118	-133
30	28	13	-2	-18	-33	-48	-63	-79	-94	-109	-125	-140
35	27	11	-4	-20	-35	-51	-67	-82	-98	-113	-129	-145
40	26	10	-6	-21	-37	-53	-69	-85	-100	-116	-132	-148
	Green				Yellow			Red				
(Wind speeds greater than 40 mph have little additional effect.)	LITTLE DANGER (for properly clothed person). Maximum danger of false sense of securtiy.				INCREASING DANGER Danger from freezing of exposed flesh.			GREAT DANGER				
	Trenchfoot and immersion foot may occur at any point on this chart											

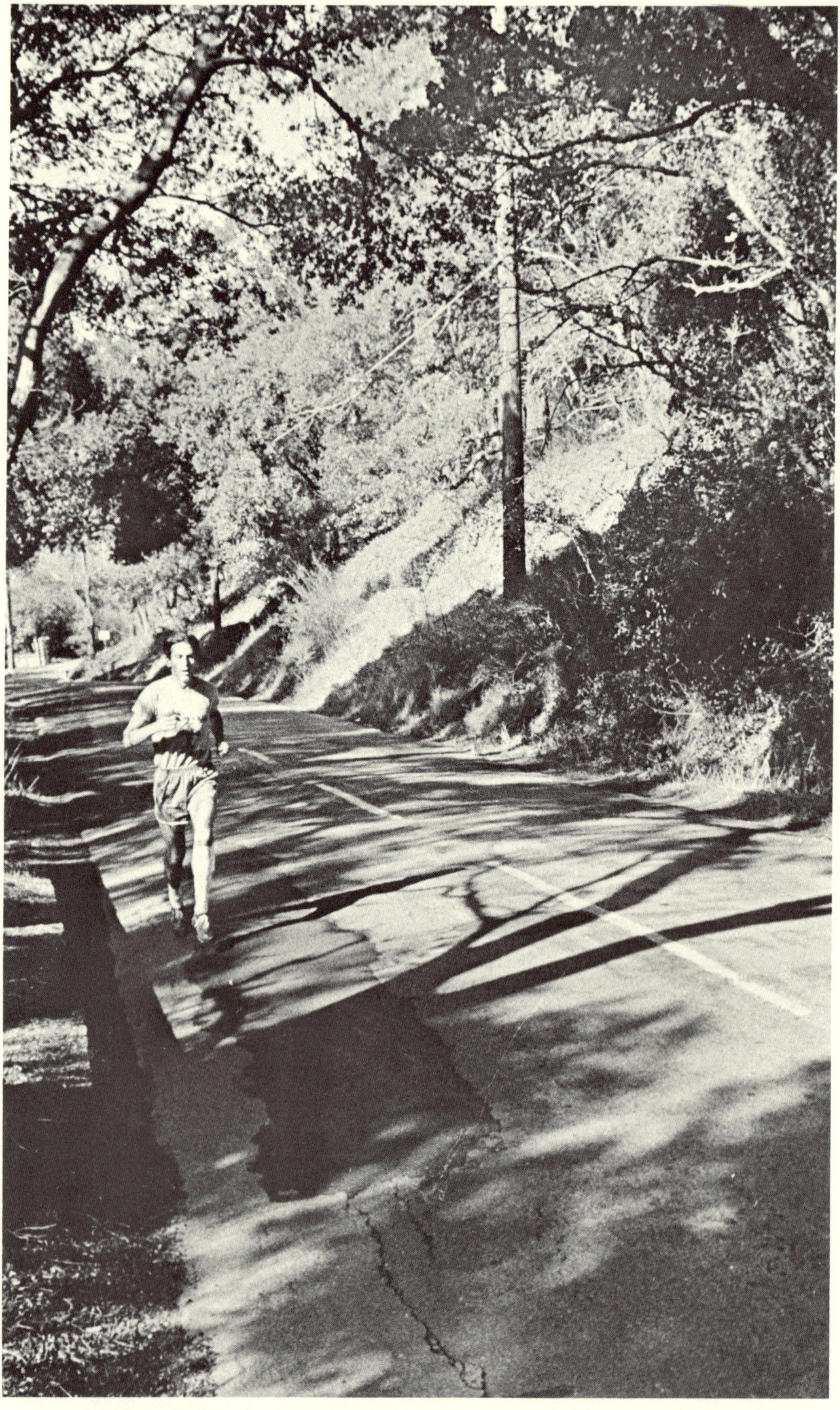

THE AIR YOU BREATHE

Many runners simply have no choice. They either run while breathing polluted air, or they don't run at all. Smoggy, dirty air is constantly with us if we live in or near most major cities.

In the Los Angeles area, school teachers are instructed to curtail unnecessary outdoor physical activity when smog reaches certain levels. Officials feel the exercise, in these conditions, would do more harm than good.

On one particularly smoggy day, athletes in 10 northern New Jersey communities became ill during practice. Their nausea, headaches, chest pains and muscle spasms were said to be directly related to "high concentrations of oxidants in the atmosphere."

When general polution counts are high, the runner simply has to weigh the potential benefits against the potential harm. He can't run away from the smog.

Exposure to carbon monoxide is of at least equal concern—especially to road runners. But in this case, he *can* run away from the heaviest concentrations.

The highest levels, naturally, are along the busiest streets. On major streets, these levels are high enough during peak traffic hours to cause a significant health hazard.

Carbon monoxide levels are measured in parts per million (ppm). Studies in major cities in the US, Europe and Japan have shown that on hot, windless days these levels reach an average of 50 ppm—and double or even triple that on the most congested streets and at stoplights. (However, a gentle wind can reduce this by 90%.)

Researchers at Stanford University have determined that a carbon monoxide exposure above 27 ppm (for one hour) can result in partial loss of vision, an impairment of judgment, and other symptoms.

Since carbon monoxide fumes—which, incidentally, are both colorless and odorless—extend as much as 65 feet on either side of the busy street, runners can only escape them by getting completely away from heavy traffic.

Asher J. Finkel of the AMA Department of Environmental Public, and Occupational Health, writes, "Jogging along a busy highway does entail a significant exposure to air pollutants that may be deleterious to health. It would certainly be preferable to jog along country lanes or lightly traveled city streets. Furthermore, there is the obvious hazard of physical contact with moving vehicles..."

References: *Environment, November 1971; Asher J. Finkel, Journal of the American Medical Association, Feb. 28, 1972; Marge Davenport, Oregon Journal, March 13, 1972.*

Page 86: Unfortunately, not all runners get to practice in surroundings like these. Country-clean air is rare. City smog tends to be the rule. (George Beinhorn photo)

ALTITUDE ADAPTATION

The environment at high altitude is characterized by the following: (1) low atmospheric oxygen pressure; (2) low air density; (3) dry air, and (4) intense solar radiation. These can affect runners, though not always negatively (in the case of sprinters and hurdlers there are compensating advantages).

There has been shown to be little or no effect when unacclimatized athletes run at elevations up to 3000 feet. Above that, altitude becomes increasingly more of a factor for these reasons:

- *Low atmospheric oxygen pressure* diminishes the athlete's maximum intake, and therefore influences sustained running pace.
- *Low air density* decreases the air resistance and makes it possible to run faster at distances where oxygen intake isn't a major consideration. (Two minutes is the approximate dividing line where altitude quits helping and begins to hurt performance.)
- *Dry air* contributes to dehydration and dryness in the nose and throat.
- *Solar radiation,* along with dry air, contributes to heat stress in long distance races.

Initial exposure to high altitude also tends to cause difficulty in getting to sleep, an increase in heart rate, occasional light-headedness, and possibly mild illnesses in the first few days. Vigorous training during the first few days and weeks at altitude can lead to excessive fatigue and stress symptoms.

When racing at high altitude, one of two courses of action is recommended: (1) race immediately after arrival; or (2) train at that level for about four weeks. The theory is that a newly-arrived runner hits his "low" several days after arriving, then gradually begins to adapt to the elevation.

Even after acclimatizing, all runners will be slower (in races 1500 meters and up) than they can run at sea level. At 7500 feet, the loss in time is estimated at 5-10 seconds per mile, or more.

Lactic acid accumulates faster than usual under these oxygen-short conditions. For this reason, hills and erratic pace take more of a toll than usual. Collapse during or after races is much more common at altitude. But no prolonged ill effects have been observed.

Chapter Five

Medical Care

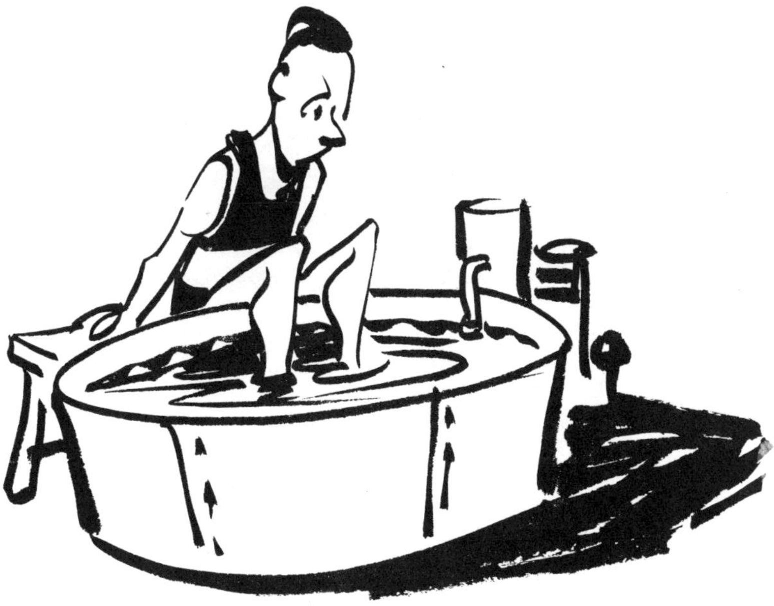

INTRODUCTION

The role of sports medicine is changing and expanding. Unfortunately, there will always be a crying need for people who approach it from the negative side: fixing broken bodies. Runners who push themselves to the limits of speed and endurance will keep going over the edge, and there must be someone there to help and advise them when they do.

But sports medicine also has a newer and more promising role. It involves the prevention of injury and illness by identifying the sources of these ailments. That's part of it. A second part is even more positive. It involves testing athletes to determine their capabilities and their limitations, to evaluate the effects of training, and to mate this knowledge to produce best possible results.

Though this testing is outside the scope of this booklet, we'd be remiss not to mention the growing part these men are playing. A number of scientists are at work around the United States and the world, and they are providing valuable data. In the US, Drs. David Costill, Kenneth Cooper, Jack Daniels, Michael Pollock, Jack Wilmore and many others have done ground-breaking studies of runners. Their work has produced several revelations that apply to training and racing methods, and at the same time they have buried some myths about what the sport does and doesn't do.

Applying running methods is still an art. But the scientist is clearly taking his place alongside the artist in the care and feeding of runners. They make a good team.

Even among the doctors testing and/or treating runners, teamwork appears to be valuable. The problems among runners are so subtle and complex that a single specialist may not be able to handle them. The best answers may come from a team composed of physician, podiatrist, physiologist, psychologist, biochemist, physiotherapist—and of course the coach and athlete.

The methods employed by the "treaters" and the "testers" differ. One uses the cast and the prescription; the other relies on the treadmill and oxygen uptake tables. But their aims are the same: to remove barriers from the athlete's path, thereby letting him go as far as his inherent ability and will allow.

THE TEAM TREATMENT

BY GEORGE SHEEHAN, M.D.

"The diseases we athletes suffer from are subtle," says Eamon O'Reilly, American marathon record holder. "But doctors treat us like battered bodies just hauled off the football field. Then when we don't improve they get frustrated and don't want us around the office any more."

O'Reilly was voicing a common complain' among athletes, and especially runners, about their present medical care. What they and the doctors are suffering from is the lost art of making a diagnosis, because medicine (as with every profession that gets into specialization) has lost its central art. It has taken it from the individual and given it to the group, the committee, or the team.

Unfortunately, even the team approach to disease has not reached the examining rooms where the athlete is treated. Sports medicine has traditionally been the province of the orthopedic surgeon, who is by temperament a man of action. His instinct is to cut, inject, or manipulate. His knowledge of total body metabolic and biochemical interrelationships is as sketchy as the medical man's grasp of skeletal stresses and strains. It makes you wonder whether any man be adequate for the job.

Perhaps not. A colleague of mine once said, "I'm a specialist because I don't know enough to be a general practioner." There were, in the old days, such generalists. They were called diagnosticians. When insoluble problems arose, they were called upon to find the thread of truth which ran through the apparently contradictory facts, to bring order out of chaos. They were distinguished by their logic, their powers of observation, but mostly by their simplicity. That was the common denominator. The solution, when arrived at, was so obvious, the wonder was that it wasn't seen right from the beginning.

What this demands is time and wisdom and a life style all out of tune with our times. The patient is willing and wanting and waiting to tell the physician the answer to his problem. But if things work out the way medical care is going, he will be telling his story to a computer. No doctor has the time to listen, to analyze, to diagnose.

A temporary solution was proposed in the *Journal of the American Medical Association* by two Canadian physicians greatly interested in sports medicine. Drs. Tom Fried and Don Shephard asked for a team approach to the athlete and his problems. Giving up on the possibility of medical schools producing a physician knowledgeable enough to care for the total athlete, they recommend that the physician, physiologist, biochemist and psychologist act as a closely knit team with such technical experts as the physical educator, the coach and the trainer.

To document their brief, the Toronto medics report four illustrative case histories: "The Runner with the Aching Legs," sidelined for a whole season until it was noticed that his arches were too high, rather than too low; the problem of the "Breathless Cyclist" whose shortness of breath was due to the fact that he keyed his breathing to his pumping action and he overbreathed on hills; the mystery of the "Asthmatic Swimmer"–it was due to the chlorine in the pool; and the enigma of the "Versatile Cyclist"—his leg cramps came from training for and racing in pursuit races and distance races at the same time. His sprint muscles then cramped up on the hills and in the endurance race.

These four cases can, I'm sure, be multipled by the thousands. There are athletes of all ages and competence being deprived of a literally essential part of their daily life because of the inadequate and superficial approach to their medical care.

I doubt that even the team idea will be the total solution. What we need is the attention of those great but simple and open-minded men in American medicine. We must direct the laser-like analytical powers of these men to these diseases of excellence, the illnesses of those who pursue the maximum metabolic, muscular, cardio-pulmonary and psychological steady state attainable by man.

Only from such physicians, our current generalists, will we find that sports medicine embraces the study of man from Anatomy to Zen. Only they will tell us the obvious—that resilience, grace and integrity of the body from foot to brow are necessary. Podiatry and Modern Dance may mean more than cortisone and the scalpel.

No disease would be too subtle for that team.

ROAD TO RECOVERY

Knowing you should "rest" an injury or illness and actually laying off to allow recovery are entirely different matters.

Patience is a virtue in the treatment of any ailment. But it isn't a trait that runners seem to have in great supply. As soon as they're back on their feet, they're wanting to run again. At this point, they're prime candidates for a repeat performance.

Inactivity bothers a runner. He not only fears falling behind his competitors, but long-term running also seems to produce a psychological and physical dependence on regular exercise.

Frederick Baekeland set out to study the reactions of steady exercisers to deprivation of their exercise. He used observations of their sleep patterns.

First Finding: Difficulty in getting volunteers. Steady exercisers refused to participate despite the offer of a stipend. Many asserted that they would not stop exercising for any amount of money. As a result, he could not obtain daily exercisers to do experiments. He finally settled for three-day-a-week athletes.

Second Finding: During the month of exercise deprivation, these subjects developed an impairment of sleep patterns which indicated anxiety. They also had increased tension and an increased need to be with others.

This study helps us understand why runners feel lousy when they can't run. It also suggests a course of rehabilitation that takes these facts into account.

The athlete who is forced to stop running must make every effort to:

1. *Maintain his cardio-pulmonary condition.*
2. *Maintain strength, endurance and flexibility in his muscles.*
3. *Avoid weight gain.*
4. *Minimize the attendant depression.*

One answer is to substitute an activity which is at the same time (a) safe; (b) physically beneficial; (c) psychologically satisfying. Three substitues are particularly good in this regard:

- **Swimming**—An excellent cardiopulmonary conditioner. It will not detract from strength gained through other training programs, and contributes to endurance and flexibility of muscles used. *One mile of swimming equals four miles of running.*

- **Bicycling**—If tolerated, it can provide cardiopulmonary conditioning along with excellent training for legs. It can be done either outdoors on the roads or indoors on a stationary cycle. *Four miles of cycling equals one mile of running.*

- **Weight Training**—Selective strength, endurance and flexibility exercises can be done. When used with swimming, weights give a balanced program for the injured athlete.

In the absence of training, deconditioning occurs at about the following rate: (a) speed suffers if you go five or more days without speed training; (b) endurance declines if you go over a week without distance work.

You should keep in mind, too, that a break for hard racing and competition can sometimes be a blessing as well. Injury and disability can remove the the athlete from a situation that was too much for him to begin with. In such instances, the rest may provide much needed therapy.

References: *Frederick Baekeland, Archives of General Psychiatry, April 1970; Practical Running Psychology, May 1970; George Sheehan, Runner's World, March 1972.*

AILMENTS — 'A' TO 'Z'

The original idea was to organize this like a conventional encyclopedia—in alphabetical order. But no sooner had we started than we realized this was impossible—because the human body isn't organized in alphabetical order. It operates as interrelated systems. So the booklet generally follows the lines of these systems. This alphabetical chart helps you find information fast about specific subjects.